LIPEDEMA
DIET COOKBOOK
FOR BEGINNERS

Delicious and Nutritious Recipes with Expert Guidance to Manage Symptoms, Enhance Well-Being, and Support Your Journey to Health

Kingsley Klopp

To show our appreciation for your purchase, we're delighted to offer you these special bonuses as a heartfelt thank you

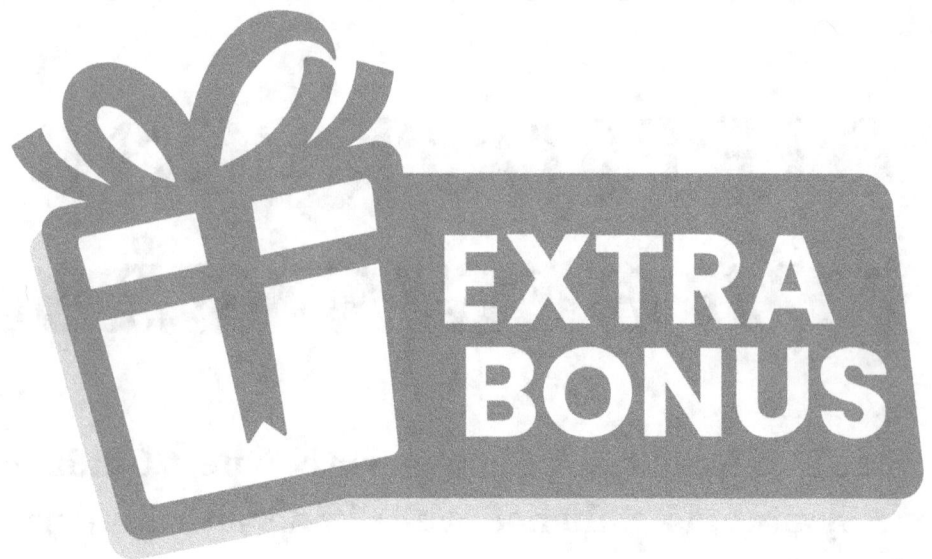

1. A Food Tracker Journal
2. Downloadable E-BOOK featuring full-color images of finished recipes

Copyright © 2024 All rights reserved.

No part of this book may be reproduced or transmitted in any form or by any means, electronic or mechanical, including photocopying, recording, or by any information storage and retrieval system, without written permission from the author. The scanning, uploading, and distribution of this book via the internet or via any other means without the permission of the author is illegal and punishable by law. The author has made every effort to ensure the accuracy of the information contained in this book. However, the author cannot be held responsible for any errors or omissions.

Table of Content

Introduction..7

Chapter 1: Understanding Lipedema
- What is Lipedema?...9
- Causes and Symptoms...11
- Diagnosis and Stages...13
- Treatment Options..15

Chapter 2: Lipedema-Friendly Diet Principles
- Anti-inflammatory Foods..18
- Importance of Hydration...21
- Foods to Avoid...24

Breakfast Recipes

Oatmeal with Walnuts...26
Spinach and Mushroom Omelette..27
Greek Yogurt Parfait..28
Almond Flour Pancakes..29
Buckwheat Porridge..30
Turkey Sausage Scramble..31
Quinoa Breakfast Bowl...32
Kale and Tomato Frittata...33
Vegan Tofu Scramble..34
Sweet Potato Hash..35
Pumpkin Oatmeal..36
Millet Porridge...37
Egg Muffins...38
Zucchini Bread..39
Savory Quinoa Bowl..40
Kefir with Berries...41
Almond Butter Smoothie...41
Bircher Muesli..42

Turkey and Spinach Crepes..43
Berry and Chia Yogurt..44
Flaxseed and Banana Muffins..45
Lentil Salad with Poached Eggs..46
Baked Cod with Olives and Tomatoes..47

Vegetables Recipes
Roasted Brussels Sprouts with Garlic..48
Kale and Quinoa Salad..49
Zucchini Noodles with Pesto..50
Butternut Squash Risotto...51
Spinach and Feta Stuffed Mushrooms...52
Grilled Eggplant with Tomato and Basil..53
Green Bean Almondine...54
Roasted Turnips with Parsley..55
Stir-fried Bok Choy..56
Vegetarian Chili..57
Asparagus Lemon Pasta...58
Cabbage Slaw with Honey Lime Dressing...59
Sautéed Swiss Chard with Pine Nuts...60
Spaghetti Squash Primavera...61
Roasted Radishes with Rosemary..62
Eggplant Caponata..63

Poultry Recipes
Grilled Chicken Salad..64
Turkey Chili..65
Chicken Stir-fry...66
Roasted Turkey Breast..67
Chicken Zoodle Soup...68
Baked Chicken Thighs with Dijon Mustard...69
Turkey Meatballs in Marinara Sauce..70
Chicken Stuffed Bell Peppers...71
Herb-Roasted Turkey Legs...72
Chicken and Spinach Curry..73
Turkey Lettuce Wraps..74
Chicken and Vegetable Kebabs...75
Buffalo Chicken Salad..76
Turkey and Sweet Potato Hash..77
Chicken Caprese...78
Asian Turkey Meatloaf...79
Turkey and Spinach Stuffed Shells...80

Chicken Fajitas...81
Turkey and Cabbage Stir-fry..82
Balsamic Glazed Chicken Breast..83
Pesto Turkey Pinwheels..84
Roasted Chicken with Root Vegetables...85
Smoked Paprika Turkey Legs...86
Chicken Bruschetta...87
Chicken and Asparagus Stir-fry...88
Lemon and Thyme Turkey Cutlets..89

Fish Recipes
Grilled Salmon with Lemon and Herbs..90
Baked Cod with Olive Tapenade..91
Asian-Inspired Tuna Poke Bowl...92
Sardines in Tomato Sauce..93
Herb-Crusted Tilapia...94
Mackerel Salad...95
Trout Almondine..96
Spicy Grilled Shrimp..97
Lemon Butter Haddock..98
Salmon and Quinoa Salad..99
Halibut Steaks with Mango Salsa..100
Sea Bass with Fennel and Orange...101
Smoked Salmon Frittata...102
Panko-Crusted Sole...103
Scallops with Pea Puree..104
Barramundi with Lemon Caper Sauce...105
Stuffed Trout with Spinach and Pine Nuts..106
 Grilled Mackerel with Herb Salad..107
Pan-Seared Tuna Steaks...108
Broiled Snapper with Tomato Relish..109
Cajun Catfish with Sweet Potato Mash..110
Shrimp and Asparagus Stir-fry..111
Mediterranean Baked Sardines...112
Flounder with Parsley Sauce..113
Scallop and Chorizo Paella...114
Anchovy and Green Bean Salad..115
Honey Glazed Salmon..116

Soup& Stew Recipes
Lentil and Spinach Soup...117
Split Pea Soup..118

White Bean and Kale Soup..119
Thai Coconut Shrimp Soup...120
Miso Soup with Tofu..121
Vegetable Beef Stew...122
Chicken Tortilla Soup..123
Barley and Mushroom Soup...124
Spicy Black Bean Soup..125
Italian Sausage and Potato Soup..126
Sweet Potato and Red Lentil Soup..127
Caribbean Chicken Stew...128

10-WEEK MEAL PLAN..**129**

Important Note

As you set out on this culinary adventure, we want to remind you that each individual's dietary needs can be quite unique, particularly for those managing lipedema.

While the recipes in this cookbook are crafted to provide balanced and nutritious meals, it's important to listen to your body and make adjustments according to your specific nutritional requirements and preferences. Your health is our top priority, and we encourage you to use these recipes as a flexible guide, tailoring them to suit your personal health goals.

We strongly recommend consulting with your healthcare provider or a registered dietitian before making any significant changes to your diet. Their expert guidance will help ensure that your dietary choices are safe and effective, providing you with the best possible support on your health journey.

Please also note that the nutritional information provided for each recipe is approximate and may vary based on the specific ingredients and brands you use. While we strive to offer accurate information, variations in portion sizes and ingredient types can influence the nutritional content.

Furthermore, If our cookbook has brought joy to your kitchen and table, we'd be thrilled to hear about your experiences in an Amazon review. On the flip side, if you stumble upon any hiccups while exploring our recipes, don't hesitate to get in touch at **kloppkingsley@gmail.com.** We're here to support your cooking journey every step of the way.

Introduction

Welcome to the **Lipedema Diet Cookbook for Beginners** – your new culinary companion in the journey of managing Lipedema with flavor, flair, and a dash of empowerment! Whether you've just been diagnosed or you've been navigating this condition for years, this cookbook is crafted with you in mind, offering practical, delicious, and nutritious solutions tailored to your unique needs. Imagine a world where every meal not only tantalizes your taste buds but also supports your health and well-being. That's the world we're inviting you into – a world where the right foods can make a profound difference in how you feel every day. Lipedema, as you might know too well, is a condition that brings its challenges – from the persistent pain and swelling to the emotional rollercoaster of finding what works for you. But here's the good news: what you eat can be a powerful tool in your arsenal against these challenges.

You might be wondering, "*How can food really help?*" Well, let's break it down. Lipedema is often accompanied by chronic inflammation and fluid retention, making it crucial to focus on an anti-inflammatory diet. The recipes and tips in this book are designed to reduce inflammation, improve lymphatic function, and support your overall health. We're talking about vibrant salads bursting with color and nutrients, hearty meals that satisfy without compromising your health, and sweet treats that won't leave you feeling guilty. But this book is more than just a collection of recipes. It's a guide to understanding the role of nutrition in managing Lipedema, helping you make informed choices that align with your health goals. We'll delve into the science of anti-inflammatory foods, explore the importance of hydration, and highlight foods to avoid to keep your symptoms at bay. Our aim is to empower you with knowledge and inspire you with delicious, easy-to-make meals that fit seamlessly into your lifestyle. We know that starting something new can be daunting, especially when it comes to changing your diet. That's why we've made this cookbook as user-friendly as possible. Each recipe comes with step-by-step instructions, nutritional information, and tips to make preparation a breeze. Whether you're a kitchen novice or a seasoned home cook, you'll find that these recipes are accessible, flavorful, and packed with ingredients that love you back.

But let's be real for a moment – managing Lipedema is not just about the physical aspect; it's also about the emotional journey. Food is deeply personal and tied to our memories, cultures, and daily routines. We want to honor that connection by offering recipes that are not only nutritious but also comforting and familiar. Think of this cookbook as a friend who understands your struggles and is here to make your journey a little easier, one delicious bite at a time.

Throughout this book, you'll find stories from individuals who have transformed their lives through diet and lifestyle changes. Their journeys are a testament to the power of food as medicine and a reminder that you're not alone in this. You'll also find practical tips for meal planning, grocery shopping, and dining out, ensuring that you can maintain your healthy eating habits no matter where life takes you.

So, let's set out on this flavorful adventure together. Open these pages with an open heart and a curious palate. Allow yourself to explore new ingredients, try new recipes, and discover how nourishing your body with the right foods can bring a new sense of vitality and well-being. The **Lipedema Diet Cookbook for Beginners** is here to support you, inspire you, and celebrate every small victory along the way.

Chapter 1: Understanding Lipedema
What is Lipedema?

Lipedema, a term that many are unfamiliar with, is a chronic disorder affecting millions of women worldwide, yet it remains shrouded in mystery and often misunderstood. This condition is not just about the physical changes it brings but the emotional and psychological battles it wages on those affected. To understand Lipedema, we must talk about its origins, its development over time, and its profound impact on the lives of countless individuals.

Lipedema was first described in the medical literature in the 1940s by Dr. Edgar Allen and Dr. Edgar Hines at the Mayo Clinic. They recognized a unique pattern of fat distribution that primarily affected women, causing disproportionate enlargement of the lower body. Unlike typical obesity, Lipedema fat accumulates symmetrically on the legs, thighs, hips, and sometimes arms, while the feet and hands remain unaffected. This distribution often results in a distinctive, column-like appearance of the legs, earning Lipedema the nickname *"painful fat syndrome."* The origins of Lipedema are still not fully understood, but it is believed to have a strong genetic component. Many women with Lipedema have a family history of the condition, suggesting an inherited predisposition. Hormonal changes, particularly those associated with puberty, pregnancy, and menopause, seem to trigger or exacerbate the condition, which may explain why Lipedema predominantly affects women.

Lipedema's development is insidious and relentless. It often begins during puberty or other hormonal shifts, with the first signs appearing as subtle swelling or a feeling of heaviness in the legs. Over time, the fat deposits become more pronounced, leading to a noticeable discrepancy between the upper and lower body. The skin overlying the affected areas may become tender and bruises easily, adding to the physical discomfort. As Lipedema progresses, it can have a profound impact on mobility and quality of life. The excessive fat deposits can make walking and physical activity challenging, leading to a sedentary lifestyle and further exacerbating the condition. Many women with Lipedema describe a feeling of being trapped in their own bodies, their movements restricted by the weight they carry.

Beyond the physical burden, Lipedema carries a heavy emotional toll. Society often misunderstands or dismisses the condition as simple obesity, leading to feelings of shame, frustration, and isolation. Women with Lipedema frequently encounter healthcare professionals who are unaware of the condition or misdiagnose it, compounding their sense of helplessness. The lack of awareness and understanding can make it difficult for those affected to find the support and treatment they need.

However, the story of Lipedema is not one of despair alone. In recent years, there has been a growing movement to raise awareness and improve the lives of those living with the condition. Advocacy groups, researchers, and medical professionals are working tirelessly to educate the public, develop effective treatments, and provide a sense of community for those affected. Living with Lipedema requires immense strength and resilience. It is a journey of self-discovery and self-acceptance, of finding ways to manage the condition and reclaim one's life. For many women, connecting with others who share their experiences can be a lifeline, offering validation and support in a world that often fails to understand.

In summary, Lipedema is a complex and challenging condition that affects millions of women worldwide. Its origins may be rooted in genetics and hormonal changes, but its impact reaches far beyond the physical. The journey of living with Lipedema is one of perseverance, courage, and hope. By raising awareness and fostering understanding, we can create a more compassionate and supportive environment for those affected by this often-misunderstood condition. Together, we can help illuminate the path towards better treatments, greater acceptance, and a brighter future for all those living with Lipedema.

Causes and Symptoms of Lipedema

Causes of Lipedema

1. *Genetic Predisposition*: One of the primary factors contributing to Lipedema is genetics. Many women with Lipedema report a family history of the condition, indicating that it may be inherited. Researchers believe that certain genetic mutations could predispose individuals to developing Lipedema. However, the specific genes involved have yet to be fully identified, and more research is needed to pinpoint the genetic markers.

2. *Hormonal Influences*: Hormonal changes play a significant role in the onset and progression of Lipedema. The condition often manifests during periods of hormonal fluctuation, such as puberty, pregnancy, and menopause. This pattern suggests that estrogen and other hormones may influence the distribution and storage of fat in individuals with Lipedema. Hormonal changes can trigger the initial appearance of symptoms or exacerbate existing ones.

3. *Inflammatory Factors*: Some studies suggest that Lipedema may be associated with chronic inflammation. The abnormal fat cells in Lipedema patients are thought to release inflammatory substances that contribute to the swelling and tenderness characteristic of the condition. This inflammation can further damage lymphatic vessels, leading to secondary lymphedema in advanced stages.

4. *Microvascular Dysfunction*: Emerging research points to the possibility of microvascular dysfunction in individuals with Lipedema. This means that the small blood vessels in the affected areas may not function properly, leading to increased permeability and fluid leakage. This vascular dysfunction could contribute to the abnormal fat accumulation and the tendency for the skin to bruise easily.

5. *Unknown Environmental Triggers*: While genetics and hormonal changes are significant factors, environmental triggers may also play a role in Lipedema. These could include lifestyle factors, dietary habits, and other environmental exposures. However, the exact nature of these triggers remains unclear, and further research is needed to understand how they might interact with genetic and hormonal factors to cause Lipedema.

Symptoms of Lipedema

The symptoms of Lipedema can vary widely among individuals, but they typically follow a recognizable pattern. The progression of symptoms can be gradual, making early detection challenging. Here are the key symptoms associated with Lipedema:

1. *Symmetrical Fat Accumulation*: One of the hallmark symptoms of Lipedema is the symmetrical accumulation of fat in the legs, thighs, hips, and sometimes the arms. This fat distribution creates a characteristic appearance, often described as a "column-like" or "tree-trunk" shape. The feet and hands are usually spared, which helps distinguish Lipedema from other conditions like obesity.

2. *Pain and Tenderness*: The fat deposits in Lipedema are often painful to the touch. Individuals with Lipedema may experience tenderness, aching, and a feeling of heaviness in the affected areas. This pain can be persistent and significantly impact daily activities and overall quality of life.

3. *Easy Bruising*: The skin overlying the affected areas is typically more prone to bruising. Even minor trauma or pressure can cause significant bruising, which can be distressing for those with Lipedema. This symptom is a result of the fragile nature of the blood vessels in the affected fat tissue.

4. *Swelling*: Swelling, or edema, is a common symptom of Lipedema. This swelling is not caused by fluid retention but rather by the abnormal fat cells and the inflammatory processes associated with the condition. The swelling can worsen throughout the day, particularly after prolonged periods of standing or sitting.

5. *Reduced Mobility*: As Lipedema progresses, the increased fat deposits and swelling can limit mobility. Walking and physical activities may become more challenging, leading to a sedentary lifestyle. This reduction in activity can further exacerbate the condition, creating a vicious cycle.

6. *Emotional and Psychological Impact*: The physical symptoms of Lipedema are often accompanied by significant emotional and psychological challenges. The changes in body shape and the chronic pain can lead to feelings of self-consciousness, depression, and anxiety. Many individuals with Lipedema struggle with body image issues and social isolation due to the visible and painful nature of the condition.

7. *Secondary Lymphedema*: In advanced stages, Lipedema can lead to secondary lymphedema, a condition where the lymphatic system becomes compromised, causing additional swelling. This occurs because the lymphatic vessels are damaged by the chronic inflammation and abnormal fat accumulation, leading to a buildup of lymph fluid.

Diagnosis and Stages of Lipedema

Diagnosis of Lipedema

Diagnosing Lipedema can be challenging due to its overlapping symptoms with other conditions such as obesity and lymphedema. However, a thorough clinical evaluation, patient history, and specific diagnostic criteria can help in accurately identifying Lipedema.

1. Clinical Evaluation: The first step in diagnosing Lipedema involves a detailed clinical evaluation by a healthcare professional familiar with the condition. The evaluation typically includes:
- Physical Examination: A physical examination focuses on the characteristic symmetrical fat distribution in the legs, thighs, hips, and sometimes the arms, while sparing the feet and hands. The presence of pain, tenderness, and easy bruising in these areas is also assessed.
- Patient History: A thorough patient history is taken to understand the onset and progression of symptoms, family history of Lipedema or similar conditions, and any previous diagnoses or treatments.

2. Diagnostic Criteria: Specific diagnostic criteria for Lipedema have been established to aid in its identification. These criteria include:
- Symmetrical Fat Distribution: The fat accumulation is typically symmetrical, affecting both sides of the body equally.
- Sparing of Hands and Feet: Unlike lymphedema, Lipedema does not affect the hands and feet, which remain unaffected and are a key distinguishing feature.
- Pain and Tenderness: Affected areas are often painful and tender to the touch.
- Easy Bruising: The skin over the affected areas bruises easily due to the fragility of blood vessels.
- Hormonal Influences: Symptoms often appear or worsen during periods of hormonal change, such as puberty, pregnancy, or menopause.

3. Differential Diagnosis: Differentiating Lipedema from other conditions with similar presentations is crucial. This involves ruling out:
- Obesity: Unlike generalized obesity, Lipedema fat is resistant to diet and exercise, and the distribution is distinctively disproportionate.
- Lymphedema: Lymphedema involves fluid retention and swelling in the limbs, including the hands and feet, and may develop secondary to Lipedema in advanced stages.
- Chronic Venous Insufficiency: This condition can cause swelling and skin changes but does not exhibit the same pattern of fat distribution as Lipedema.

4. Imaging Studies: While not always necessary, imaging studies such as ultrasound, MRI, or lymphoscintigraphy can be used to assess the extent of fat tissue and rule out other conditions. These studies can provide detailed information about the structure of the affected tissues.

Stages of Lipedema

Lipedema progresses through distinct stages, each with its own characteristics and implications for treatment. Recognizing these stages helps in planning appropriate management strategies.

Stage 1: Early Lipedema
- Characteristics: The skin remains smooth, but there is an increase in fatty tissue, particularly in the hips, thighs, and buttocks. Patients may notice a feeling of heaviness and pain in the legs, along with easy bruising.
- Implications: Early intervention is crucial at this stage to manage symptoms and slow progression. Lifestyle changes, compression therapy, and exercise can be beneficial.

Stage 2: Moderate Lipedema
- Characteristics: The skin begins to develop an uneven texture with a nodular appearance due to the formation of small lumps in the fatty tissue. The affected areas become more sensitive and painful.
- Implications: More intensive treatments may be needed, including manual lymphatic drainage, compression garments, and potentially surgical interventions such as liposuction to remove excess fat.

Stage 3: Advanced Lipedema
- Characteristics: The skin becomes hard and uneven, with larger lumps and more pronounced fatty deposits. The affected limbs may take on a column-like appearance, and mobility can be significantly impaired.
- Implications: Management focuses on reducing symptoms, improving mobility, and preventing complications. Surgical options may be more commonly considered at this stage, and ongoing physical therapy is often necessary.

Stage 4: Lipolymphedema
- Characteristics: In this advanced stage, Lipedema is often accompanied by secondary lymphedema, where the lymphatic system is damaged, leading to additional swelling and fluid retention.
- Implications: Treatment becomes more complex and may involve a combination of lymphatic drainage, compression therapy, and surgical interventions. Managing secondary lymphedema is critical to prevent further complications.

Importance of Early Diagnosis and Intervention

Early diagnosis and intervention are vital in managing Lipedema effectively. Recognizing the condition in its initial stages allows for timely implementation of treatments that can slow its progression, alleviate symptoms, and improve quality of life. Awareness and education among healthcare professionals and the public are essential to ensure that Lipedema is identified and treated appropriately.

Treatment Options for Lipedema

Non-Surgical Treatments
1. Compression Therapy: Compression therapy is a cornerstone in the management of Lipedema. It involves wearing compression garments such as stockings, leggings, or sleeves that apply consistent pressure to the affected areas. This pressure helps reduce swelling, improve lymphatic flow, and alleviate pain. Compression garments should be fitted by a professional to ensure proper size and effectiveness.
2. Manual Lymphatic Drainage (MLD): MLD is a specialized massage technique designed to stimulate the lymphatic system and promote the drainage of lymph fluid. This therapy can help reduce swelling, pain, and the feeling of heaviness in the limbs. MLD should be performed by a trained therapist familiar with Lipedema and its unique requirements.
3. Exercise and Physical Activity: Regular exercise is crucial for managing Lipedema, as it helps improve lymphatic flow, maintain a healthy weight, and enhance overall mobility. Low-impact exercises such as swimming, walking, cycling, and water aerobics are particularly beneficial. Exercise routines should be tailored to individual capabilities and monitored by healthcare professionals to prevent injury and overexertion.
4. Healthy Diet and Nutrition: A balanced diet can help manage symptoms and improve overall health. Although diet alone cannot cure Lipedema, it can play a supportive role in treatment. Anti-inflammatory diets rich in fruits, vegetables, lean proteins, and healthy fats are recommended. Reducing the intake of processed foods, sugars, and unhealthy fats can help control inflammation and support weight management.
5. Psychological Support and Counseling: The emotional impact of Lipedema can be profound, leading to feelings of frustration, depression, and social isolation. Psychological support through counseling or support groups can help individuals cope with the emotional challenges of living with Lipedema. Connecting with others who share similar experiences can provide invaluable support and encouragement.

Medical and Pharmacological Treatments
1. Lipedema-Specific Supplements: Certain supplements, such as horse chestnut extract, omega-3 fatty acids, and antioxidants, may help reduce inflammation and improve symptoms. However, these should be used under the guidance of a healthcare professional to ensure safety and effectiveness.
2. Anti-Inflammatory Medications: In some cases, anti-inflammatory medications may be prescribed to help manage pain and reduce inflammation. These medications should be used as part of a comprehensive treatment plan and monitored for potential side effects.

Surgical Treatments

For many individuals with Lipedema, especially in the more advanced stages, surgical intervention may be necessary to remove excess fat deposits and improve quality of life. The following surgical options are commonly used:

1. Liposuction: Liposuction is the most effective surgical treatment for Lipedema. It involves the removal of fat deposits through small incisions using a cannula. There are several techniques of liposuction used in Lipedema treatment:

- Tumescent Liposuction: This technique involves injecting a large volume of a diluted local anesthetic solution into the fatty tissue before removing it. This method helps minimize bleeding and swelling.
- Water-Assisted Liposuction (WAL): This technique uses a jet of water to dislodge and remove fat cells. It is gentle on the tissues and can be effective in reducing pain and recovery time.
- Lymph-Sparing Liposuction: This specialized technique aims to preserve the lymphatic vessels while removing fat deposits. It is particularly important in preventing further complications such as lymphedema.

Liposuction can significantly reduce pain, improve mobility, and enhance the overall appearance of the affected limbs. However, it is not a cure for Lipedema, and ongoing management with non-surgical treatments is necessary to maintain results.

2. Bariatric Surgery: While bariatric surgery is not a primary treatment for Lipedema, it may be considered in cases where the individual also has severe obesity. Weight loss from bariatric surgery can help reduce the strain on the lymphatic system and improve overall health. However, it is important to note that Lipedema fat is resistant to diet and exercise, so this surgery will not specifically target Lipedema fat deposits.

Emerging Treatments and Research

Research into Lipedema is ongoing, and new treatments are continually being explored. Some emerging treatments include:

1. Stem Cell Therapy: Stem cell therapy is being investigated as a potential treatment for Lipedema. This therapy involves the use of stem cells to regenerate and repair damaged tissues, potentially improving lymphatic function and reducing inflammation. However, this treatment is still in the experimental stages, and more research is needed to determine its safety and efficacy.

2. Laser Therapy: Laser therapy is another emerging treatment that may help reduce fat deposits and improve lymphatic flow. It involves the use of targeted laser energy to break down fat cells and stimulate the lymphatic system. This therapy is still under investigation and should be considered experimental at this stage.

3. Nutraceuticals and Pharmacotherapy: Research is also focusing on the development of nutraceuticals and pharmaceutical agents that can target the underlying mechanisms of Lipedema, such as inflammation and fat metabolism. These treatments hold promise but are not yet widely available.

Comprehensive Management Approach

Effectively managing Lipedema requires a comprehensive, multidisciplinary approach that combines various treatment modalities. Collaboration among healthcare providers, including physicians, physical therapists, dietitians, and mental health professionals, is essential to provide holistic care.

1. Personalized Treatment Plans: Treatment plans should be tailored to the individual's specific needs, considering the stage of Lipedema, overall health, and personal preferences. Regular follow-up and adjustments to the treatment plan are necessary to address changing symptoms and needs.

2. Patient Education: Educating patients about Lipedema, its progression, and available treatments is crucial for empowering them to take an active role in their care. Understanding the condition helps patients make informed decisions and adhere to their treatment plans.

3. Support Networks: Building a support network, including family, friends, and support groups, can provide emotional and practical support. Connecting with others who share similar experiences can offer encouragement and reduce feelings of isolation.

Chapter 2: Lipedema-Friendly Diet Principles
Anti-inflammatory Foods

Lipedema is a chronic condition marked by the abnormal accumulation of fat, predominantly in the lower body, accompanied by pain, tenderness, and easy bruising. One of the critical components of managing Lipedema is adopting an anti-inflammatory diet. Chronic inflammation plays a significant role in the progression of Lipedema, and incorporating anti-inflammatory foods can help mitigate symptoms, reduce inflammation, and improve overall health.

The Importance of Anti-inflammatory Foods
Chronic inflammation is a hallmark of Lipedema, exacerbating pain, swelling, and the overall progression of the condition. Anti-inflammatory foods help combat this inflammation, providing relief from symptoms and supporting the body's natural healing processes. These foods are rich in antioxidants, vitamins, minerals, and healthy fats, which collectively contribute to reducing inflammation and promoting overall well-being.

Key Anti-inflammatory Foods
1. Fruits and Vegetables: Fruits and vegetables are the cornerstone of an anti-inflammatory diet due to their high content of antioxidants, vitamins, and minerals. They help neutralize free radicals and reduce oxidative stress, which is linked to inflammation.

- Berries: Blueberries, strawberries, raspberries, and blackberries are packed with antioxidants and vitamins, particularly vitamin C, which help reduce inflammation.
- Leafy Greens: Spinach, kale, Swiss chard, and arugula are rich in vitamins A, C, E, and K, as well as fiber and antioxidants, making them powerful anti-inflammatory foods.
- Cruciferous Vegetables: Broccoli, cauliflower, Brussels sprouts, and cabbage contain sulforaphane, an antioxidant that has been shown to reduce inflammation.
- Tomatoes: Tomatoes are high in lycopene, an antioxidant that helps combat inflammation and protect against chronic diseases.

2. Healthy Fats: Incorporating healthy fats into the diet is crucial for reducing inflammation. These fats provide essential fatty acids that the body cannot produce on its own.
- Olive Oil: Extra virgin olive oil is rich in monounsaturated fats and polyphenols, which have strong anti-inflammatory properties. It can be used in cooking, salad dressings, and as a finishing oil.
- Fatty Fish: Salmon, mackerel, sardines, and trout are excellent sources of omega-3 fatty acids, which have been shown to reduce inflammation and support heart health.
- Avocados: Avocados are high in monounsaturated fats, fiber, and antioxidants, making them a nutritious and anti-inflammatory addition to the diet.
- Nuts and Seeds: Walnuts, almonds, chia seeds, and flaxseeds provide omega-3 fatty acids and other nutrients that help reduce inflammation.

3. Whole Grains: Whole grains are rich in fiber, which helps regulate blood sugar levels and reduce inflammation. Unlike refined grains, whole grains retain their nutrients and provide sustained energy.
- Quinoa: Quinoa is a gluten-free whole grain that is high in protein, fiber, and various vitamins and minerals. It is an excellent alternative to refined grains.
- Brown Rice: Brown rice is a whole grain that provides fiber, magnesium, and other nutrients that support overall health and reduce inflammation.
- Oats: Oats are a great source of soluble fiber, which helps lower cholesterol levels and reduce inflammation. They can be enjoyed as oatmeal, in smoothies, or as a base for homemade granola.

4. Lean Proteins: Lean proteins support muscle maintenance and repair without contributing to inflammation. They are an essential part of a balanced diet for individuals with Lipedema.
- Poultry: Chicken and turkey are excellent sources of lean protein. Opt for skinless, white meat cuts to reduce saturated fat intake.
- Legumes: Beans, lentils, and chickpeas are plant-based sources of protein and fiber. They provide essential nutrients and help reduce inflammation.
- Tofu and Tempeh: These soy-based products are high in protein and can be used in various dishes as meat alternatives.

5. Herbs and Spices: Herbs and spices not only add flavor to dishes but also possess potent anti-inflammatory properties.
- Turmeric: Turmeric contains curcumin, a compound with powerful anti-inflammatory and antioxidant effects. It can be added to curries, soups, and smoothies.
- Ginger: Ginger has been shown to reduce inflammation and pain. It can be used fresh, dried, or in supplement form.
- Garlic: Garlic is known for its anti-inflammatory and immune-boosting properties. It can be used in a variety of savory dishes.
- Cinnamon: Cinnamon has anti-inflammatory and antioxidant effects. It can be added to oatmeal, smoothies, and baked goods.

6. Hydrating Foods: Staying well-hydrated is crucial for managing Lipedema, and certain foods can help maintain proper hydration.
- Cucumber: Cucumbers have a high water content and are low in calories, making them an excellent hydrating food.
- Watermelon: Watermelon is another hydrating fruit that provides vitamins A and C, which support overall health and reduce inflammation.
- Celery: Celery is low in calories and high in water content, making it a refreshing and hydrating snack.

Importance of Hydration

The Role of Hydration in the Body
Water is vital for numerous bodily functions, including:
- Cellular Functions: Water is essential for cellular activities, including nutrient absorption, waste removal, and energy production.
- Temperature Regulation: Sweating and respiration help regulate body temperature, both of which rely on adequate hydration.
- Joint Lubrication: Synovial fluid, which cushions and lubricates joints, is composed primarily of water.
- Digestive Health: Water aids in digestion, nutrient absorption, and bowel regularity, preventing constipation.
- Circulatory Health: Blood is over 90% water, and adequate hydration ensures proper circulation, delivering oxygen and nutrients to cells.

Hydration and Lipedema
For individuals with Lipedema, maintaining proper hydration is particularly important due to the following reasons:

1. Lymphatic System Support: The lymphatic system, responsible for removing waste and toxins from the body, plays a crucial role in managing Lipedema. Adequate hydration ensures that lymph fluid flows smoothly, reducing the risk of blockages and promoting efficient waste removal. When the body is dehydrated, lymph fluid can become thicker and more difficult to circulate, exacerbating swelling and discomfort.

2. Reducing Swelling and Edema: Swelling and edema are common symptoms of Lipedema. Proper hydration can help reduce these symptoms by promoting fluid balance and preventing fluid retention. When the body is well-hydrated, it is less likely to retain excess fluids, which can otherwise accumulate in the tissues and cause swelling.

3. Improving Skin Health: Individuals with Lipedema often experience skin issues, including dryness and easy bruising. Staying hydrated helps maintain skin elasticity and integrity, reducing the risk of skin breakdown and irritation. Well-hydrated skin is more resilient and can better withstand the physical changes associated with Lipedema.

4. Enhancing Digestion and Nutrient Absorption: Proper hydration supports digestive health by aiding in the breakdown and absorption of nutrients. For individuals with Lipedema, a nutrient-rich diet is essential for managing inflammation and supporting overall health. Water helps transport these nutrients to cells and tissues where they are needed.

5. Supporting Weight Management: Hydration plays a role in weight management by supporting metabolism and reducing appetite. Drinking water before meals can help create a sense of fullness, preventing overeating. Additionally, proper hydration can enhance metabolic processes, supporting a healthy weight which is crucial for managing Lipedema symptoms.

Practical Tips for Maintaining Hydration

Maintaining proper hydration requires conscious effort, especially for individuals with Lipedema. Here are some practical tips to ensure adequate hydration:

1. Drink Plenty of Water: Aim to drink at least 8-10 glasses (about 2-2.5 liters) of water per day. This amount can vary based on individual needs, activity levels, and environmental factors. Listen to your body's thirst signals and drink water regularly throughout the day.

2. Eat Hydrating Foods: Incorporate hydrating foods into your diet, such as fruits and vegetables with high water content. Examples include cucumbers, watermelon, oranges, strawberries, and leafy greens. These foods not only provide hydration but also essential vitamins and minerals.

3. Start Your Day with Water: Begin your day with a glass of water to kickstart hydration. This helps replenish fluids lost during the night and prepares your body for the day ahead.

4. Carry a Water Bottle: Keep a reusable water bottle with you at all times. This makes it easy to drink water throughout the day, whether you're at work, exercising, or running errands. Set reminders if necessary to ensure you drink water regularly.

5. Monitor Your Hydration Status: Pay attention to signs of dehydration, such as dark urine, dry mouth, headache, and fatigue. Aim for light yellow urine as an indicator of proper hydration. If you notice symptoms of dehydration, increase your water intake.

6. Limit Diuretics: Reduce the consumption of diuretics such as caffeine and alcohol, as they can increase fluid loss and contribute to dehydration. If you do consume these beverages, balance them with additional water intake.

7. Flavor Your Water: If you find plain water unappealing, try adding natural flavors. Infuse water with slices of lemon, lime, cucumber, or fresh herbs like mint and basil. This can make drinking water more enjoyable and encourage you to drink more.

8. Hydrate During Physical Activity: Exercise can increase fluid loss through sweat. Ensure you drink water before, during, and after physical activity to stay properly hydrated. For intense or prolonged exercise, consider electrolyte-replenishing drinks to maintain fluid balance.

Hydration Myths and Facts

It's important to distinguish between hydration myths and facts to make informed decisions about water intake:

Myth: You can drink too much water.Fact: While it is possible to drink excessive amounts of water, leading to a condition called water intoxication or hyponatremia, it is rare and typically occurs in extreme circumstances. For most people, drinking the recommended daily amount of water poses no risk.

Myth: Thirst is the best indicator of hydration.Fact: Thirst is a late indicator of dehydration. By the time you feel thirsty, your body may already be mildly dehydrated. It's important to drink water regularly, even before you feel thirsty.

Myth: All fluids hydrate equally.Fact: While water is the best source of hydration, other fluids can contribute to your daily intake. However, sugary and caffeinated beverages can have diuretic effects and should not replace water as your primary hydration source.

Foods to Avoid for Managing Lipedema

The Impact of Inflammatory Foods on Lipedema
Foods that promote inflammation can aggravate Lipedema symptoms, including pain, swelling, and the progression of fat accumulation. These foods often contain high levels of refined sugars, unhealthy fats, and artificial additives, which can lead to increased inflammation and worsen overall health. By avoiding these foods, individuals with Lipedema can help reduce inflammation, manage symptoms, and improve their quality of life.

Foods to Avoid
1. Refined Carbohydrates and Sugars: Refined carbohydrates and sugars are among the most inflammatory foods. They can lead to rapid spikes in blood sugar levels, promote fat storage, and increase inflammation.

- Sugary Beverages: Sodas, energy drinks, and sugary fruit juices are high in refined sugars and can significantly contribute to inflammation and weight gain. Opt for water, herbal teas, or infused water instead.
- Processed Sweets: Candies, cakes, cookies, and pastries are loaded with refined sugars and unhealthy fats. These treats should be consumed sparingly, if at all.
- White Bread and Pasta: Made from refined grains, these foods lack fiber and essential nutrients. Choose whole grain or alternative grain options like quinoa or brown rice instead.
- Breakfast Cereals: Many commercial cereals are high in sugar and refined grains. Look for whole grain, low-sugar options or opt for homemade granola.

2. Trans Fats and Saturated Fats: Trans fats and excessive saturated fats are known to promote inflammation and should be avoided to manage Lipedema effectively.

- Fried Foods: Foods like French fries, fried chicken, and doughnuts are typically cooked in unhealthy oils containing trans fats. Choose baked or grilled options instead.
- Margarine and Shortening: These products often contain trans fats. Use healthier alternatives like olive oil or avocado oil.
- Processed Meats: Sausages, hot dogs, and bacon are high in saturated fats and preservatives. Opt for lean, unprocessed meats and plant-based proteins.
- High-Fat Dairy Products: Full-fat milk, cheese, and butter can contribute to inflammation. Choose low-fat or plant-based dairy alternatives.

3. **Processed and Packaged Foods:** Processed and packaged foods often contain a combination of refined sugars, unhealthy fats, and artificial additives that can worsen inflammation and overall health.
- Snack Foods: Chips, crackers, and pretzels are typically high in refined grains, unhealthy fats, and sodium. Choose whole food snacks like nuts, seeds, or fresh fruit.
- Frozen Meals: Many frozen meals are high in sodium, preservatives, and unhealthy fats. Preparing meals from fresh ingredients is a healthier option.
- Instant Noodles: These are high in refined carbs, unhealthy fats, and sodium. Opt for whole grain noodles or pasta made from alternative grains.

4. **High-Sodium Foods:** Excessive sodium intake can lead to water retention and increased swelling, which can exacerbate Lipedema symptoms.
- Canned Soups and Vegetables: These often contain high levels of sodium. Choose low-sodium versions or make homemade soups and use fresh or frozen vegetables.
- Processed Meats: As mentioned earlier, processed meats are not only high in unhealthy fats but also in sodium. Opt for fresh, lean meats.
- Condiments and Sauces: Many condiments and sauces, like soy sauce, ketchup, and salad dressings, are high in sodium. Use herbs, spices, and homemade dressings to add flavor.

5. **Artificial Additives and Preservatives:** Artificial additives and preservatives can contribute to inflammation and should be minimized in the diet.
- Artificial Sweeteners: Aspartame, sucralose, and other artificial sweeteners can cause digestive issues and inflammation in some individuals. Natural sweeteners like stevia or honey are better alternatives.
- Colorings and Flavorings: Artificial colorings and flavorings found in candies, sodas, and processed foods can promote inflammation. Opt for natural, whole foods instead.

6. **Alcohol:** While moderate alcohol consumption might not have significant adverse effects for everyone, it can promote inflammation and interfere with proper hydration, which is crucial for managing Lipedema.
- High-Sugar Cocktails: Cocktails mixed with sugary sodas and syrups can contribute to inflammation and weight gain. If consuming alcohol, opt for wine or spirits mixed with soda water and a splash of citrus.
- Excessive Consumption: Regular excessive alcohol intake can lead to chronic inflammation and other health issues. Moderation is key.

Breakfast Recipes

1. Oatmeal with Walnuts
Serves: 2
Cooking Time: 10 minutes
Ingredients:
- 1 cup rolled oats
- 2 cups water or unsweetened almond milk
- 1/2 teaspoon cinnamon
- 1/4 cup chopped walnuts
- 1 tablespoon chia seeds
- 1/2 cup fresh berries (blueberries, raspberries, or strawberries)
- 1 tablespoon maple syrup or honey (optional)
- 1/2 teaspoon vanilla extract

Instructions:
1. In a medium saucepan, bring the water or almond milk to a boil.
2. Stir in the rolled oats and reduce heat to low.
3. Cook for 5-7 minutes, stirring occasionally, until the oats are tender and the liquid is absorbed.
4. Add cinnamon and vanilla extract, stirring to combine.
5. Remove from heat and divide the oatmeal into two bowls.
6. Top each serving with chopped walnuts, chia seeds, fresh berries, and a drizzle of maple syrup or honey if desired.

Nutrition Information (per serving):
- Calories: 300
- Protein: 8g
- Carbohydrates: 45g
- Dietary Fiber: 8g
- Sugars: 10g
- Fat: 12g
- Saturated Fat: 1g
- Sodium: 5mg

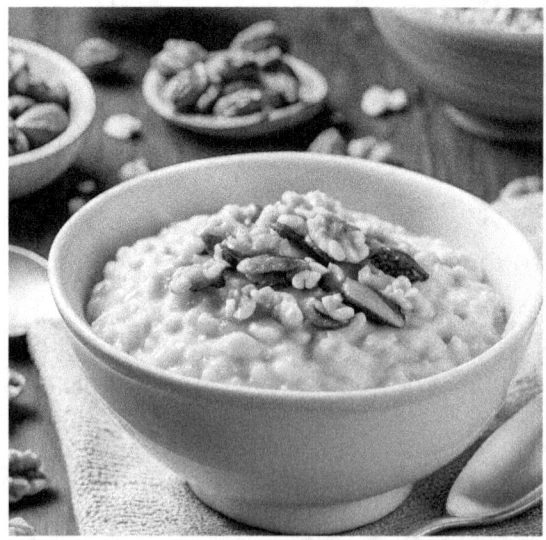

2. Spinach and Mushroom Omelette

Serves: 2
Cooking Time: 15 minutes
Ingredients:

- 4 large eggs
- 1/4 cup unsweetened almond milk
- 1 cup fresh spinach, chopped
- 1/2 cup mushrooms, sliced
- 1/4 cup diced red bell pepper
- 2 tablespoons olive oil
- 1/4 cup shredded mozzarella cheese
- 1/4 teaspoon garlic powder
- 1/4 teaspoon onion powder

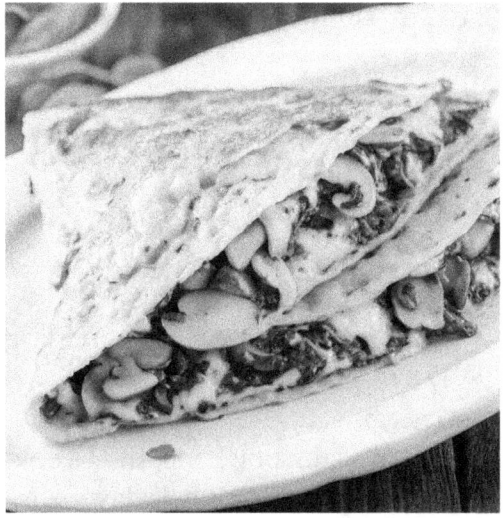

Instructions:

1. In a medium bowl, whisk together the eggs, almond milk, garlic powder, and onion powder until well combined.
2. Heat 1 tablespoon of olive oil in a non-stick skillet over medium heat.
3. Add the mushrooms and red bell pepper to the skillet, sautéing until tender, about 4-5 minutes.
4. Add the spinach to the skillet and cook until wilted, about 1-2 minutes.
5. Remove the vegetables from the skillet and set aside.
6. Add the remaining 1 tablespoon of olive oil to the skillet.
7. Pour half of the egg mixture into the skillet, cooking until the edges begin to set, about 1-2 minutes.
8. Add half of the vegetable mixture and half of the cheese to one side of the omelette.
9. Fold the other half of the omelette over the filling and cook for another 1-2 minutes until the eggs are fully cooked.
10. Repeat with the remaining egg mixture and vegetables to make the second omelette.

Nutrition Information (per serving):

- Calories: 280
- Protein: 16g
- Carbohydrates: 5g
- Dietary Fiber: 2g
- Sugars: 2g
- Fat: 22g
- Saturated Fat: 6g
- Sodium: 200mg

3. Greek Yogurt Parfait

Serves: 2

Cooking Time: 5 minutes

Ingredients:
- 2 cups plain Greek yogurt
- 1/2 cup granola (low-sugar, whole grain)
- 1/2 cup fresh berries (blueberries, raspberries, or strawberries)
- 2 tablespoons chia seeds
- 1 tablespoon honey or maple syrup (optional)
- 1/2 teaspoon vanilla extract

Instructions:
1. In a medium bowl, mix the Greek yogurt with the vanilla extract.
2. In two glasses or bowls, layer the yogurt, granola, and fresh berries.
3. Sprinkle each parfait with 1 tablespoon of chia seeds.
4. Drizzle with honey or maple syrup if desired.
5. Serve immediately.

Nutrition Information (per serving):
- Calories: 320
- Protein: 20g
- Carbohydrates: 40g
- Dietary Fiber: 7g
- Sugars: 15g
- Fat: 10g
- Saturated Fat: 2g
- Sodium: 100mg

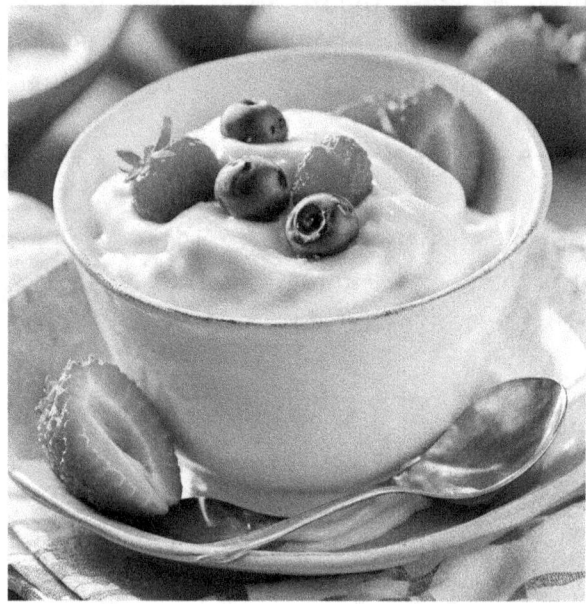

4. Almond Flour Pancakes

Serves: 2
Cooking Time: 20 minutes
Ingredients:

- 1 cup almond flour
- 2 large eggs
- 1/4 cup unsweetened almond milk
- 1 tablespoon maple syrup or honey
- 1/2 teaspoon baking powder
- 1/2 teaspoon vanilla extract
- 1/4 teaspoon cinnamon
- 1 tablespoon coconut oil (for cooking)

Instructions:

1. In a medium bowl, whisk together the almond flour, baking powder, and cinnamon.
2. In another bowl, beat the eggs and mix in the almond milk, maple syrup or honey, and vanilla extract.
3. Combine the wet and dry ingredients, mixing until smooth.
4. Heat the coconut oil in a non-stick skillet over medium heat.
5. Pour 1/4 cup of the batter onto the skillet for each pancake.
6. Cook until bubbles form on the surface and the edges are set, about 2-3 minutes.
7. Flip and cook for another 2-3 minutes until golden brown.
8. Repeat with the remaining batter.
9. Serve warm with fresh berries or a drizzle of maple syrup.

Nutrition Information (per serving):

- Calories: 350
- Protein: 14g
- Carbohydrates: 14g
- Dietary Fiber: 4g
- Sugars: 7g
- Fat: 28g
- Saturated Fat: 6g
- Sodium: 180mg

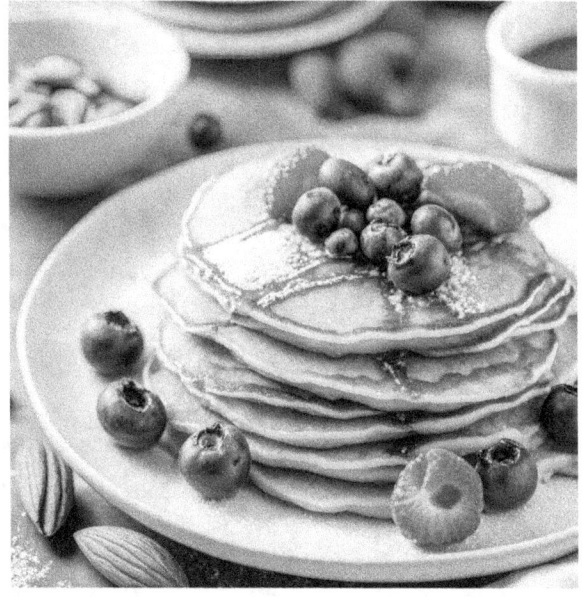

5. Buckwheat Porridge

Serves: 2
Cooking Time: 20 minutes
Ingredients:
- 1 cup buckwheat groats
- 2 cups water or unsweetened almond milk
- 1/2 teaspoon cinnamon
- 1/4 teaspoon nutmeg
- 1 tablespoon chia seeds
- 1/4 cup chopped almonds
- 1/2 cup fresh berries (blueberries, raspberries, or strawberries)
- 1 tablespoon maple syrup or honey (optional)
- 1/2 teaspoon vanilla extract

Instructions:
1. Rinse the buckwheat groats under cold water.
2. In a medium saucepan, bring the water or almond milk to a boil.
3. Add the buckwheat groats, reduce heat to low, and simmer for about 15 minutes, stirring occasionally, until the groats are tender and the liquid is absorbed.
4. Stir in the cinnamon, nutmeg, and vanilla extract.
5. Remove from heat and divide the porridge into two bowls.
6. Top each serving with chia seeds, chopped almonds, fresh berries, and a drizzle of maple syrup or honey if desired.

Nutrition Information (per serving):
- Calories: 320
- Protein: 9g
- Carbohydrates: 45g
- Dietary Fiber: 10g
- Sugars: 12g
- Fat: 12g
- Saturated Fat: 1g
- Sodium: 5mg

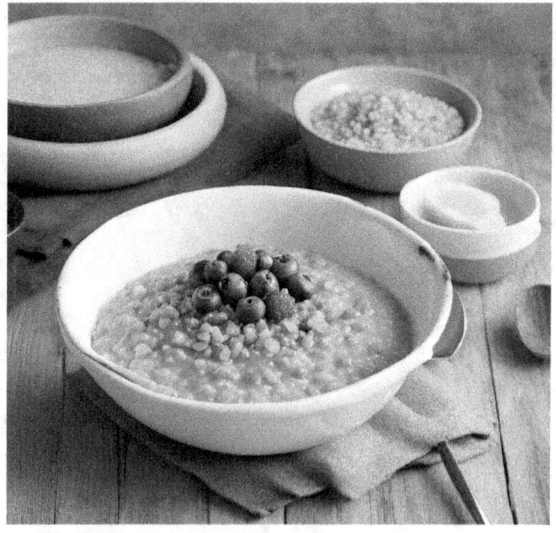

6. Turkey Sausage Scramble

Serves: 2
Cooking Time: 15 minutes
Ingredients:
- 4 large eggs
- 1/4 cup unsweetened almond milk
- 1/2 cup ground turkey sausage (low sodium)
- 1/2 cup diced bell pepper
- 1/2 cup diced onion
- 1 cup fresh spinach, chopped
- 1 tablespoon olive oil
- 1/4 teaspoon garlic powder
- 1/4 teasp

Instructions
1. In a me... powder, and paprika.
2. Heat oliv
3. Add the ... he sausage is browned
4. Add the ...
5. Pour the ... the eggs are fully coo
6. Serve im

Nutrition In
- Calories:
- Protein:
- Carbohy
- Dietary F
- Sugars: 2
- Fat: 20g
- Saturate
- Sodium:

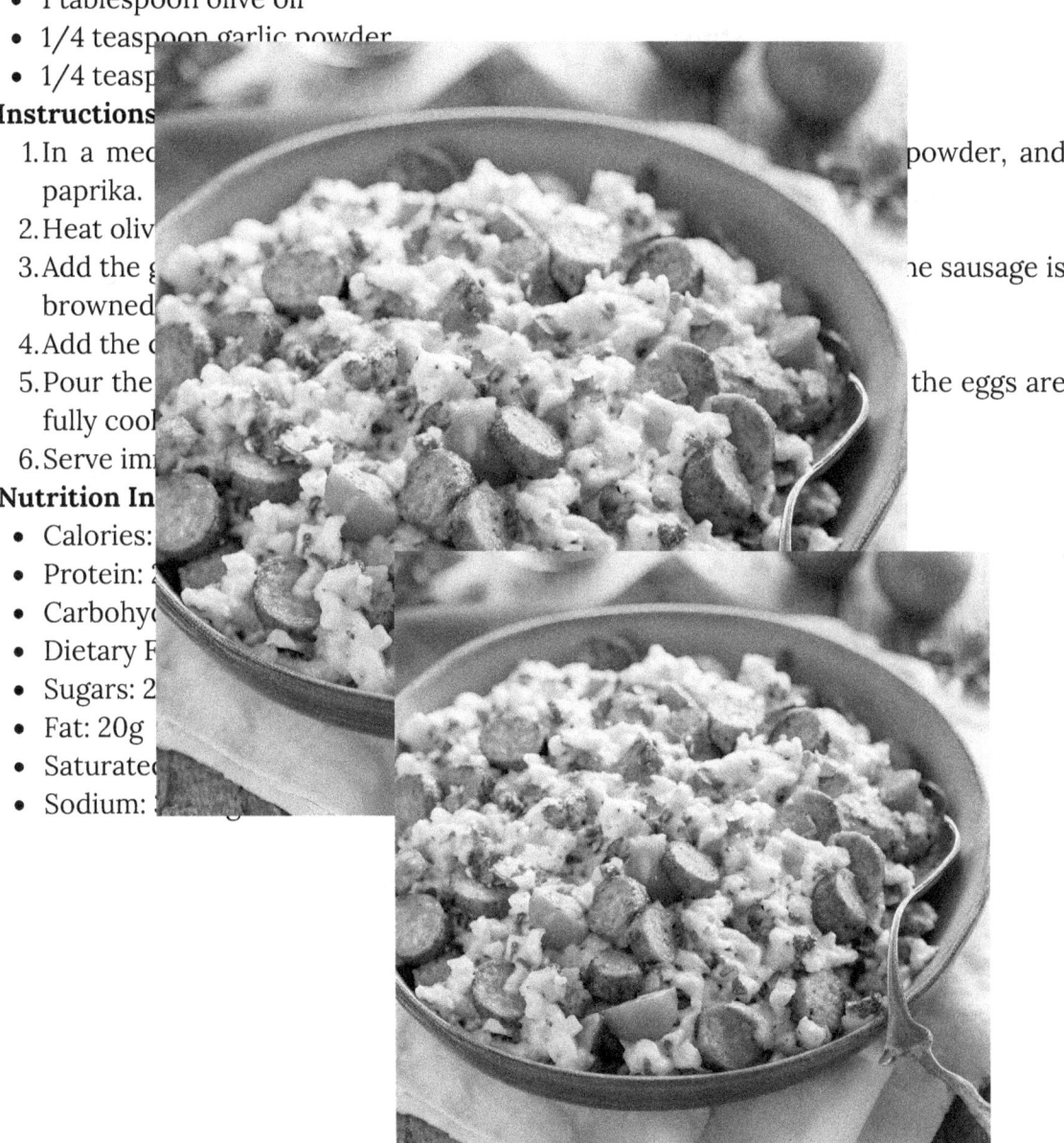

7. Quinoa Breakfast Bowl

Serves: 2
Cooking Time: 20 minutes
Ingredients:
- 1 cup cooked quinoa
- 1/2 cup unsweetened almond milk
- 1/2 teaspoon cinnamon
- 1 tablespoon chia seeds
- 1/4 cup chopped walnuts
- 1/2 cup fresh berries (blueberries, raspberries, or strawberries)
- 1 tablespoon maple syrup or honey (optional)
- 1/2 teaspoon vanilla extract

Instructions:
1. In a medium saucepan, combine cooked quinoa and almond milk. Heat over medium heat until warm, about 3-4 minutes.
2. Stir in the cinnamon, chia seeds, and vanilla extract.
3. Divide the quinoa mixture into two bowls.
4. Top each bowl with chopped walnuts, fresh berries, and a drizzle of maple syrup or honey if desired.
5. Serve warm.

Nutrition Information (per serving):
- Calories: 340
- Protein: 10g
- Carbohydrates: 45g
- Dietary Fiber: 8g
- Sugars: 10g
- Fat: 15g
- Saturated Fat: 1.5g
- Sodium: 10mg

8. Kale and Tomato Frittata

Serves: 2
Cooking Time: 25 minutes
Ingredients:
- 4 large eggs
- 1/4 cup unsweetened almond milk
- 1 cup fresh kale, chopped
- 1/2 cup cherry tomatoes, halved
- 1/4 cup diced onion
- 1/4 cup shredded mozzarella cheese
- 1 tablespoon olive oil
- 1/4 teaspoon garlic powder
- 1/4 teaspoon dried oregano

Instructions:
1. Preheat the oven to 375°F (190°C).
2. In a medium bowl, whisk together the eggs, almond milk, garlic powder, and dried oregano.
3. Heat olive oil in an oven-safe skillet over medium heat.
4. Add the diced onion and cook until tender, about 3-4 minutes.
5. Add the kale and cherry tomatoes, cooking until the kale is wilted, about 2-3 minutes.
6. Pour the egg mixture over the vegetables in the skillet.
7. Sprinkle the shredded mozzarella cheese evenly over the top.
8. Transfer the skillet to the preheated oven and bake for 10-12 minutes, or until the frittata is set and lightly golden.
9. Let cool slightly before slicing and serving.

Nutrition Information (per serving):
- Calories: 250
- Protein: 18g
- Carbohydrates: 7g
- Dietary Fiber: 2g
- Sugars: 3g
- Fat: 18g
- Saturated Fat: 5g
- Sodium: 220mg

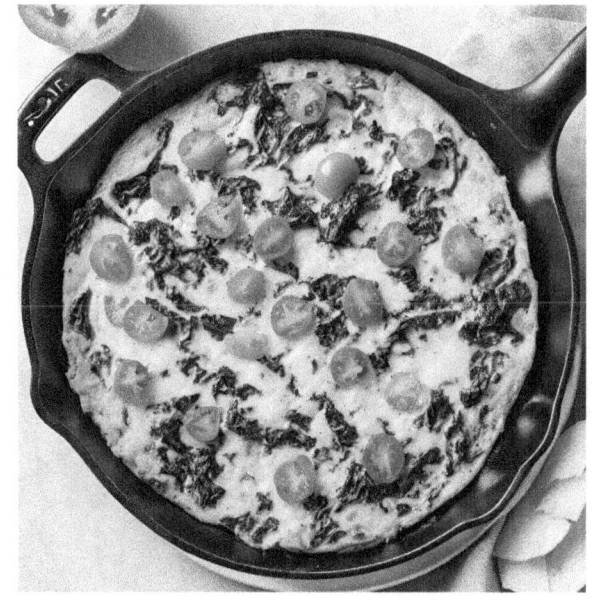

9. Vegan Tofu Scramble

Serves: 2
Cooking Time: 15 minutes
Ingredients:
- 1 block (14 oz) firm tofu, drained and crumbled
- 1/2 cup diced onion
- 1/2 cup diced red bell pepper
- 1 cup fresh spinach, chopped
- 1 tablespoon olive oil
- 1/4 teaspoon turmeric
- 1/4 teaspoon cumin
- 1/4 teaspoon garlic powder
- 1/4 teaspoon smoked paprika

Instructions:
1. Heat olive oil in a large skillet over medium heat.
2. Add the diced onion and red bell pepper, sautéing until tender, about 5 minutes.
3. Add the crumbled tofu to the skillet, stirring to combine.
4. Sprinkle the turmeric, cumin, garlic powder, and smoked paprika over the tofu mixture. Stir well to evenly coat.
5. Cook for about 5-7 minutes, stirring occasionally, until the tofu is heated through and slightly browned.
6. Add the chopped spinach and cook until wilted, about 1-2 minutes.
7. Serve immediately.

Nutrition Information (per serving):
- Calories: 220
- Protein: 18g
- Carbohydrates: 10g
- Dietary Fiber: 4g
- Sugars: 3g
- Fat: 14g
- Saturated Fat: 2g
- Sodium: 180mg

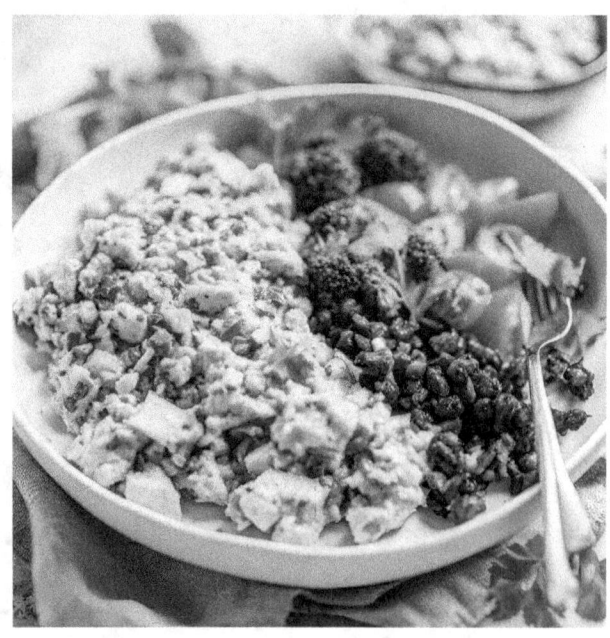

10. Sweet Potato Hash

Serves: 2
Cooking Time: 25 minutes
Ingredients:
- 2 medium sweet potatoes, peeled and diced
- 1/2 cup diced onion
- 1/2 cup diced red bell pepper
- 1/2 cup diced green bell pepper
- 2 tablespoons olive oil
- 1/4 teaspoon garlic powder
- 1/4 teaspoon smoked paprika
- 1/4 teaspoon dried thyme

Instructions:
1. Heat olive oil in a large skillet over medium heat.
2. Add the diced sweet potatoes to the skillet and cook, stirring occasionally, for about 10 minutes.
3. Add the diced onion, red bell pepper, and green bell pepper. Continue to cook for another 10-15 minutes, until the vegetables are tender and the sweet potatoes are slightly crispy.
4. Sprinkle the garlic powder, smoked paprika, and dried thyme over the mixture. Stir well to combine.
5. Serve warm.

Nutrition Information (per serving):
- Calories: 260
- Protein: 3g
- Carbohydrates: 35g
- Dietary Fiber: 7g
- Sugars: 8g
- Fat: 12g
- Saturated Fat: 1.5g
- Sodium: 60mg

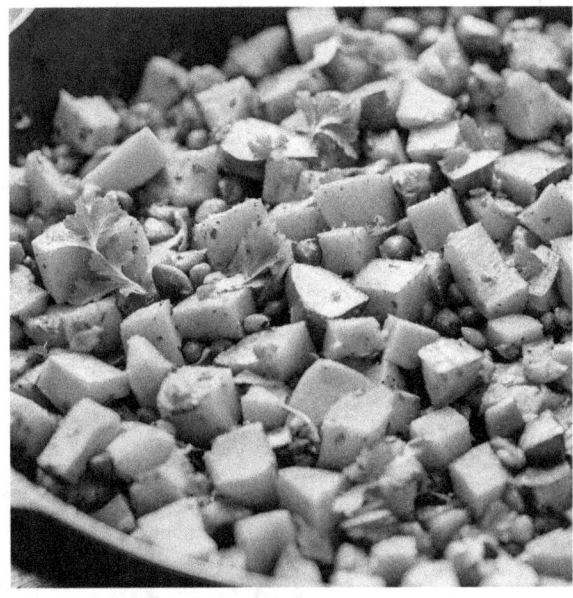

11. Pumpkin Oatmeal

Serves: 2
Cooking Time: 15 minutes

Ingredients:
- 1 cup rolled oats
- 2 cups water or unsweetened almond milk
- 1/2 cup pumpkin puree
- 1/2 teaspoon cinnamon
- 1/4 teaspoon nutmeg
- 1/4 teaspoon ginger powder
- 1 tablespoon chia seeds
- 1/4 cup chopped pecans
- 1 tablespoon maple syrup or honey (optional)
- 1/2 teaspoon vanilla extract

Instructions:
1. In a medium saucepan, bring the water or almond milk to a boil.
2. Add the rolled oats and reduce heat to low. Cook for 5-7 minutes, stirring occasionally, until the oats are tender.
3. Stir in the pumpkin puree, cinnamon, nutmeg, ginger powder, and vanilla extract. Cook for another 2-3 minutes, until heated through.
4. Remove from heat and divide the oatmeal into two bowls.
5. Top each serving with chia seeds, chopped pecans, and a drizzle of maple syrup or honey if desired.
6. Serve warm.

Nutrition Information (per serving):
- Calories: 320
- Protein: 8g
- Carbohydrates: 45g
- Dietary Fiber: 8g
- Sugars: 10g
- Fat: 12g
- Saturated Fat: 1.5g
- Sodium: 5mg

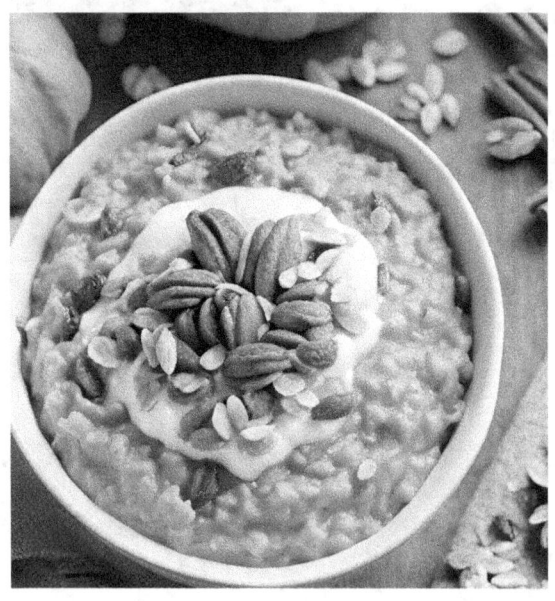

12. Millet Porridge

Serves: 2
Cooking Time: 25 minutes
Ingredients:

- 1 cup millet
- 2 cups water or unsweetened almond milk
- 1/2 teaspoon cinnamon
- 1/4 teaspoon nutmeg
- 1 tablespoon chia seeds
- 1/4 cup chopped almonds
- 1/2 cup fresh berries (blueberries, raspberries, or strawberries)
- 1 tablespoon maple syrup or honey (optional)
- 1/2 teaspoon vanilla extract

Instructions:

1. Rinse the millet under cold water.
2. In a medium saucepan, bring the water or almond milk to a boil.
3. Add the millet, reduce heat to low, and simmer for about 20 minutes, stirring occasionally, until the millet is tender and the liquid is absorbed.
4. Stir in the cinnamon, nutmeg, and vanilla extract.
5. Remove from heat and divide the porridge into two bowls.
6. Top each serving with chia seeds, chopped almonds, fresh berries, and a drizzle of maple syrup or honey if desired.
7. Serve warm.

Nutrition Information (per serving):

- Calories: 340
- Protein: 9g
- Carbohydrates: 55g
- Dietary Fiber: 8g
- Sugars: 10g
- Fat: 12g
- Saturated Fat: 1.5g
- Sodium: 5mg

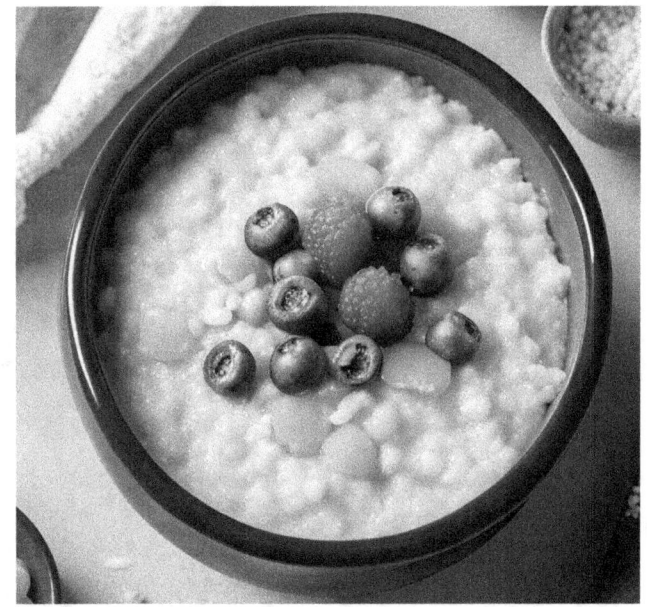

13. Egg Muffins

Serves: 6 (2 muffins per serving)
Cooking Time: 30 minutes
Ingredients:
- 8 large eggs
- 1/2 cup unsweetened almond milk
- 1 cup fresh spinach, chopped
- 1/2 cup cherry tomatoes, halved
- 1/2 cup diced red bell pepper
- 1/4 cup diced onion
- 1/4 cup shredded mozzarella cheese
- 1/4 teaspoon garlic powder
- 1/4 teaspoon dried oregano

Instructions:
1. Preheat the oven to 375°F (190°C).
2. In a large bowl, whisk together the eggs, almond milk, garlic powder, and dried oregano.
3. Add the chopped spinach, cherry tomatoes, red bell pepper, and onion to the egg mixture, stirring to combine.
4. Grease a muffin tin with a small amount of olive oil or use silicone muffin liners.
5. Pour the egg mixture evenly into the muffin cups.
6. Sprinkle shredded mozzarella cheese on top of each muffin.
7. Bake in the preheated oven for 20-25 minutes, or until the egg muffins are set and lightly golden.
8. Allow to cool slightly before removing from the muffin tin.
9. Serve warm or store in the refrigerator for up to 3 days.

Nutrition Information (per serving):
- Calories: 180
- Protein: 14g
- Carbohydrates: 5g
- Dietary Fiber: 1g
- Sugars: 2g
- Fat: 12g
- Saturated Fat: 4g
- Sodium: 180mg

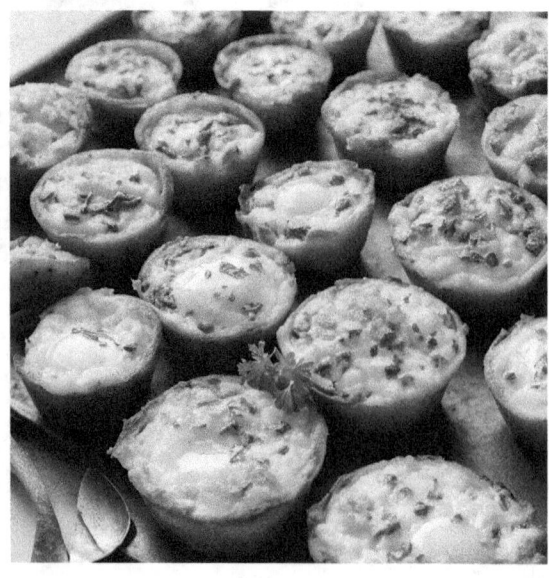

14. Zucchini Bread

Serves: 10 slices
Cooking Time: 1 hour 10 minutes
Ingredients:

- 1 1/2 cups grated zucchini
- 1 1/2 cups almond flour
- 1/2 cup coconut flour
- 1 teaspoon baking soda
- 1 teaspoon ground cinnamon
- 1/4 teaspoon ground nutmeg
- 3 large eggs
- 1/2 cup unsweetened applesauce
- 1/4 cup maple syrup or honey
- 1/4 cup olive oil
- 1 teaspoon vanilla extract
- 1/2 cup chopped walnuts

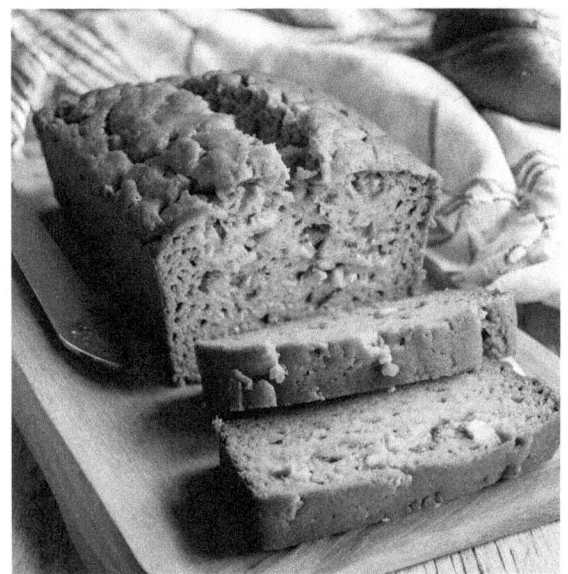

Instructions:

1. Preheat the oven to 350°F (175°C). Grease a 9x5 inch loaf pan or line it with parchment paper.
2. In a large bowl, mix the almond flour, coconut flour, baking soda, cinnamon, and nutmeg.
3. In another bowl, whisk together the eggs, applesauce, maple syrup or honey, olive oil, and vanilla extract.
4. Add the wet ingredients to the dry ingredients and mix until well combined.
5. Fold in the grated zucchini and chopped walnuts.
6. Pour the batter into the prepared loaf pan and spread it evenly.
7. Bake in the preheated oven for 50-60 minutes, or until a toothpick inserted into the center comes out clean.
8. Allow the bread to cool in the pan for 10 minutes before transferring it to a wire rack to cool completely.
9. Slice and serve.

Nutrition Information (per serving):

- Calories: 220
- Protein: 6g
- Carbohydrates: 18g
- Dietary Fiber: 4g
- Sugars: 9g
- Fat: 14g
- Saturated Fat: 2g
- Sodium: 170mg

15. Savory Quinoa Bowl

Serves: 2
Cooking Time: 25 minutes

Ingredients:
- 1 cup cooked quinoa
- 1/2 cup chickpeas, rinsed and drained
- 1/2 cup diced cucumber
- 1/2 cup cherry tomatoes, halved
- 1/4 cup diced red onion
- 1/4 cup crumbled feta cheese
- 2 tablespoons olive oil
- 1 tablespoon lemon juice
- 1/4 teaspoon garlic powder
- 1/4 teaspoon dried oregano

Instructions:
1. In a large bowl, combine the cooked quinoa, chickpeas, cucumber, cherry tomatoes, and red onion.
2. In a small bowl, whisk together the olive oil, lemon juice, garlic powder, and dried oregano.
3. Pour the dressing over the quinoa mixture and toss to combine.
4. Divide the quinoa bowl into two servings and top with crumbled feta cheese.
5. Serve immediately or refrigerate for up to 2 days.

Nutrition Information (per serving):
- Calories: 350
- Protein: 10g
- Carbohydrates: 32g
- Dietary Fiber: 6g
- Sugars: 4g
- Fat: 20g
- Saturated Fat: 5g
- Sodium: 320mg

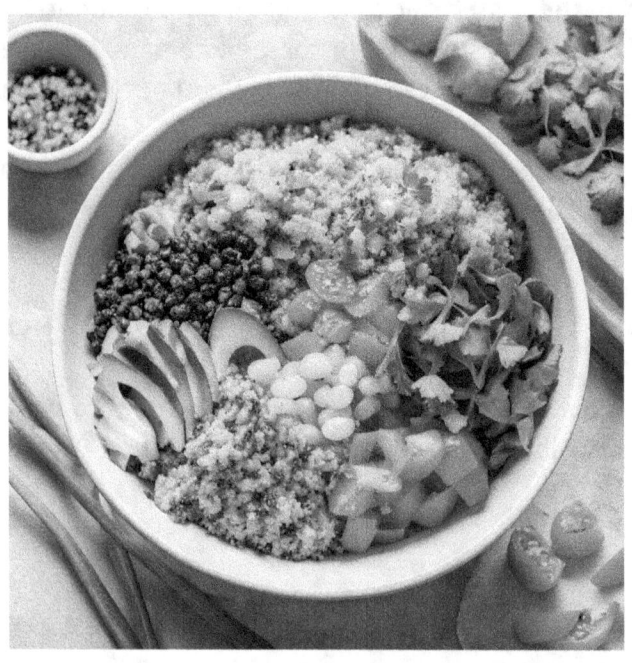

16. Kefir with Berries

Serves: 2
Cooking Time: 5 minutes
Ingredients:

- 2 cups plain kefir
- 1 cup fresh mixed berries (blueberries, raspberries, strawberries)
- 1 tablespoon chia seeds
- 1 tablespoon honey or maple syrup (optional)
- 1/2 teaspoon vanilla extract

Instructions:

1. In a medium bowl, mix the kefir with vanilla extract and honey or maple syrup if using.
2. Divide the kefir into two bowls.
3. Top each bowl with mixed berries and chia seeds.
4. Serve immediately.

Nutrition Information (per serving):

- Calories: 180 Protein: 8g Carbohydrates: 25g Dietary Fiber: 5g Sugars: 18g
- Fat: 5g
- Saturated Fat: 3g
- Sodium: 125mg

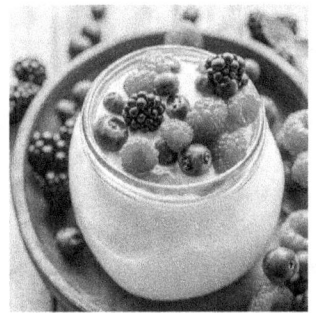

17. Almond Butter Smoothie

Serves: 2
Cooking Time: 5 minutes
Ingredients:

- 2 cups unsweetened almond milk
- 2 tablespoons almond butter
- 1 banana
- 1 tablespoon chia seeds
- 1 teaspoon vanilla extract
- 1 tablespoon honey or maple syrup (optional)
- 1/2 cup ice cubes

Instructions:

1. Combine all ingredients in a blender.
2. Blend until smooth and creamy.
3. Pour into two glasses and serve immediately.

Nutrition Information (per serving):

- Calories: 220 Protein: 5g Carbohydrates: 25g Dietary Fiber: 6g Sugars: 15g
- Fat: 12g
- Saturated Fat: 1g
- Sodium: 150mg

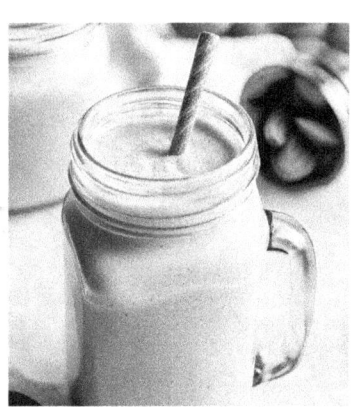

18. Bircher Muesli

Serves: 2
Cooking Time: 10 minutes (plus overnight soaking)
Ingredients:
- 1 cup rolled oats
- 1 cup unsweetened almond milk
- 1/2 cup plain Greek yogurt
- 1/2 apple, grated
- 1/4 cup chopped almonds
- 1 tablespoon chia seeds
- 1/2 teaspoon cinnamon
- 1/2 teaspoon vanilla extract
- 1 tablespoon honey or maple syrup (optional)
- 1/2 cup fresh berries (blueberries, raspberries, strawberries)

Instructions:
1. In a large bowl, mix the rolled oats, almond milk, Greek yogurt, grated apple, chopped almonds, chia seeds, cinnamon, vanilla extract, and honey or maple syrup if using.
2. Cover the bowl and refrigerate overnight.
3. In the morning, stir the mixture well.
4. Divide the muesli into two bowls and top with fresh berries.
5. Serve immediately.

Nutrition Information (per serving):
- Calories: 320
- Protein: 12g
- Carbohydrates: 45g
- Dietary Fiber: 9g
- Sugars: 15g
- Fat: 12g
- Saturated Fat: 1.5g
- Sodium: 75mg

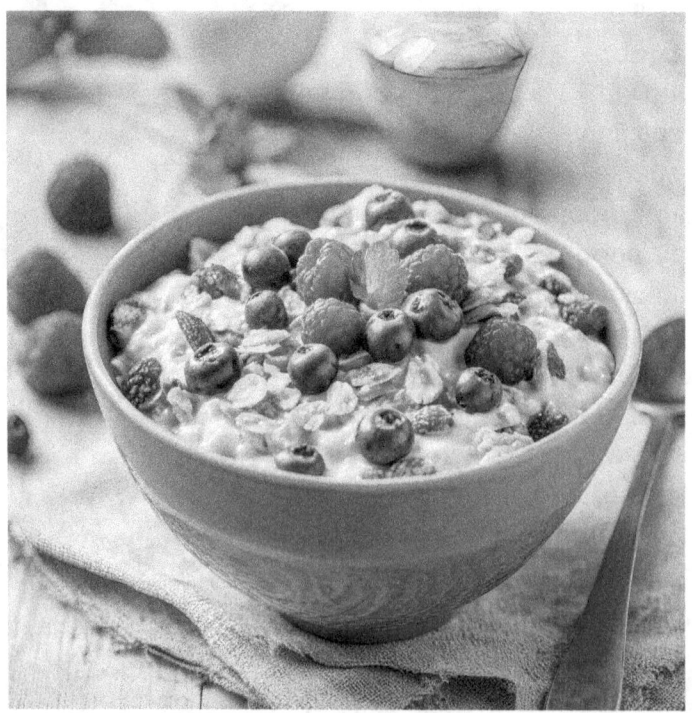

19. Turkey and Spinach Crepes

Serves: 2
Cooking Time: 30 minutes
Ingredients:

For the Crepes:
- 1 cup buckwheat flour
- 1 1/4 cups unsweetened almond milk
- 2 large eggs
- 1 tablespoon olive oil
- 1/2 teaspoon garlic powder

For the Filling:
- 1 cup cooked turkey breast, shredded
- 1 cup fresh spinach, chopped
- 1/2 cup diced tomatoes
- 1/4 cup shredded mozzarella cheese
- 1 tablespoon olive oil
- 1/4 teaspoon dried oregano

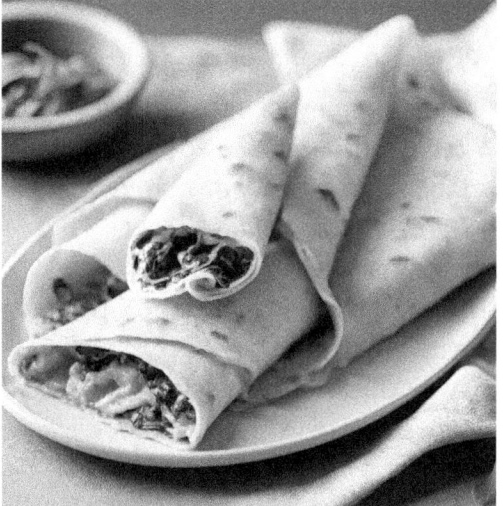

Instructions:

1. In a bowl, whisk together the buckwheat flour, almond milk, eggs, olive oil, and garlic powder until smooth.
2. Heat a non-stick skillet over medium heat. Pour in about 1/4 cup of the batter and swirl to coat the bottom of the skillet.
3. Cook for about 2 minutes, or until the edges start to lift and the crepe is lightly browned. Flip and cook for another 1-2 minutes. Remove and set aside. Repeat with the remaining batter.
4. In another skillet, heat the olive oil over medium heat. Add the shredded turkey, spinach, diced tomatoes, and dried oregano. Cook until the spinach is wilted and the turkey is heated through, about 5 minutes.
5. Place a portion of the filling in the center of each crepe, sprinkle with mozzarella cheese, fold, and serve immediately.

Nutrition Information (per serving):
- Calories: 340
- Protein: 25g
- Carbohydrates: 30g
- Dietary Fiber: 6g
- Sugars: 4g
- Fat: 14g
- Saturated Fat: 4g
- Sodium: 200mg

20. Berry and Chia Yogurt

Serves: 2
Cooking Time: 5 minutes
Ingredients:

- 2 cups plain Greek yogurt
- 1 cup mixed fresh berries (blueberries, raspberries, strawberries)
- 2 tablespoons chia seeds
- 1 tablespoon honey or maple syrup (optional)
- 1/2 teaspoon vanilla extract

Instructions:

1. In a medium bowl, mix the Greek yogurt with vanilla extract and honey or maple syrup if using.
2. Divide the yogurt into two bowls.
3. Top each bowl with mixed berries and chia seeds.
4. Serve immediately.

Nutrition Information (per serving):

- Calories: 200
- Protein: 15g
- Carbohydrates: 25g
- Dietary Fiber: 6g
- Sugars: 15g
- Fat: 5g
- Saturated Fat: 2g
- Sodium: 80mg

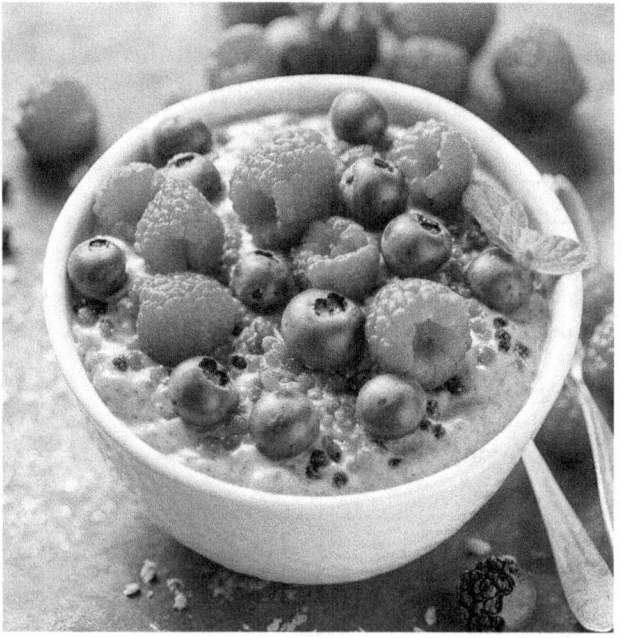

21. Flaxseed and Banana Muffins
Serves: 12 muffins
Cooking Time: 25 minutes
Ingredients:
- 1 1/2 cups almond flour
- 1/2 cup ground flaxseed
- 1 teaspoon baking soda
- 1 teaspoon ground cinnamon
- 3 large ripe bananas, mashed
- 2 large eggs
- 1/4 cup honey or maple syrup
- 1/4 cup olive oil
- 1 teaspoon vanilla extract

Instructions:
1. Preheat the oven to 350°F (175°C). Line a muffin tin with paper liners.
2. In a large bowl, mix the almond flour, ground flaxseed, baking soda, and cinnamon.
3. In another bowl, whisk together the mashed bananas, eggs, honey or maple syrup, olive oil, and vanilla extract.
4. Add the wet ingredients to the dry ingredients and mix until well combined.
5. Divide the batter evenly among the muffin cups.
6. Bake for 20-25 minutes, or until a toothpick inserted into the center comes out clean.
7. Allow to cool slightly before removing from the tin. Serve warm or at room temperature.

Nutrition Information (per muffin):
- Calories: 180
- Protein: 4g
- Carbohydrates: 20g
- Dietary Fiber: 4g
- Sugars: 10g
- Fat: 10g
- Saturated Fat: 1g
- Sodium: 90mg

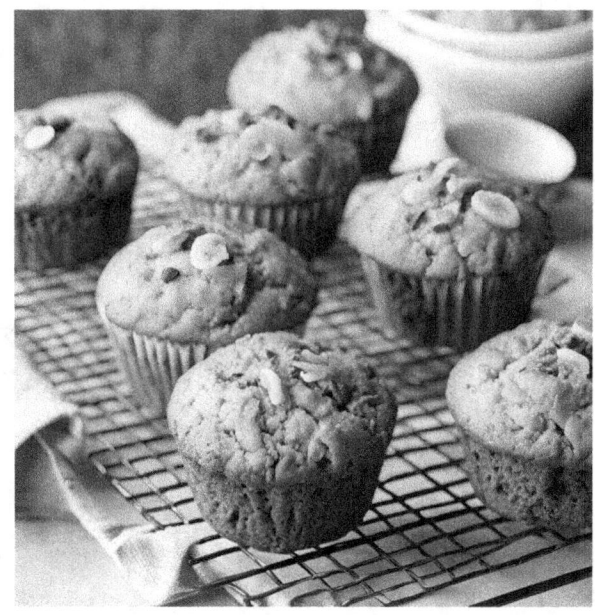

22. Lentil Salad with Poached Eggs

Serves: 2
Cooking Time: 25 minutes
Ingredients:
- 1 cup cooked lentils
- 1/2 cup diced cucumber
- 1/2 cup cherry tomatoes, halved
- 1/4 cup diced red onion
- 2 tablespoons olive oil
- 1 tablespoon lemon juice
- 1/4 teaspoon garlic powder
- 1/4 teaspoon dried thyme
- 2 large eggs
- 1 tablespoon white vinegar

Instructions:
1. In a large bowl, combine the cooked lentils, cucumber, cherry tomatoes, and red onion.
2. In a small bowl, whisk together the olive oil, lemon juice, garlic powder, and dried thyme. Pour over the lentil mixture and toss to combine.
3. To poach the eggs, bring a medium saucepan of water to a simmer. Add the white vinegar.
4. Crack each egg into a small bowl, then gently slide the eggs into the simmering water. Poach for about 3-4 minutes, until the whites are set and the yolks are still runny.
5. Remove the eggs with a slotted spoon and place them on top of the lentil salad.
6. Serve immediately.

Nutrition Information (per serving):
- Calories: 300
- Protein: 14g
- Carbohydrates: 25g
- Dietary Fiber: 10g
- Sugars: 4g
- Fat: 16g
- Saturated Fat: 3g
- Sodium: 120mg

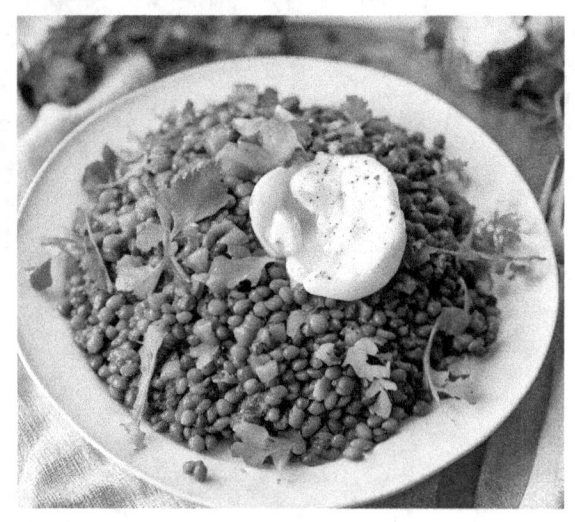

23. Baked Cod with Olives and Tomatoes

Serves: 2
Cooking Time: 30 minutes
Ingredients:
- 2 cod fillets (about 6 oz each)
- 1 cup cherry tomatoes, halved
- 1/4 cup sliced black olives
- 1/4 cup diced red onion
- 2 tablespoons olive oil
- 1/2 teaspoon dried oregano
- 1/4 teaspoon garlic powder
- 1 tablespoon lemon juice

Instructions:
1. Preheat the oven to 375°F (190°C). Line a baking dish with parchment paper.
2. Place the cod fillets in the baking dish.
3. In a bowl, combine the cherry tomatoes, black olives, red onion, olive oil, dried oregano, and garlic powder. Mix well.
4. Spoon the tomato and olive mixture over the cod fillets.
5. Drizzle with lemon juice.
6. Bake in the preheated oven for 20-25 minutes, or until the cod is opaque and flakes easily with a fork.
7. Serve immediately.

Nutrition Information (per serving):
- Calories: 280
- Protein: 30g
- Carbohydrates: 6g
- Dietary Fiber: 2g
- Sugars: 2g
- Fat: 16g
- Saturated Fat: 3g
- Sodium: 300mg

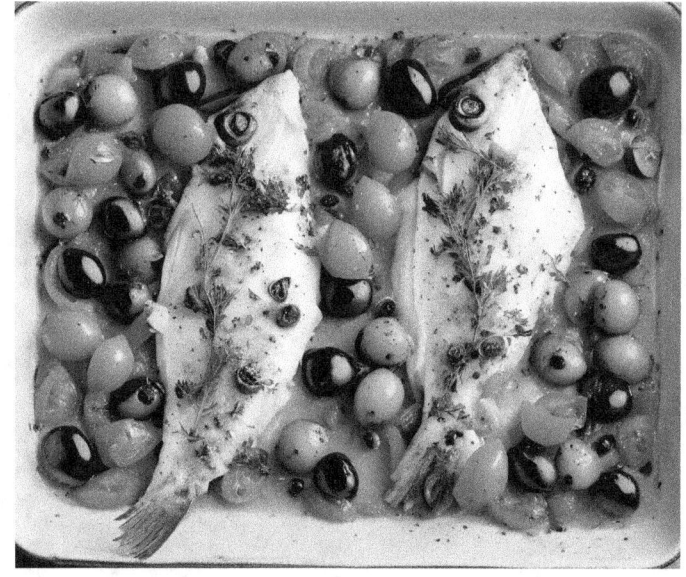

Vegetables Recipes

1. Roasted Brussels Sprouts with Garlic
Serves: 4
Cooking Time: 30 minutes
Ingredients:
- 1 1/2 pounds Brussels sprouts, trimmed and halved
- 3 tablespoons olive oil
- 4 cloves garlic, minced
- 1 teaspoon dried thyme
- 1 tablespoon lemon juice

Instructions:
1. Preheat the oven to 400°F (200°C). Line a baking sheet with parchment paper.
2. In a large bowl, toss the Brussels sprouts with olive oil, minced garlic, and dried thyme until evenly coated.
3. Spread the Brussels sprouts in a single layer on the prepared baking sheet.
4. Roast in the preheated oven for 20-25 minutes, or until the Brussels sprouts are tender and golden brown, stirring halfway through.
5. Remove from the oven and drizzle with lemon juice before serving.

Nutrition Information (per serving):
- Calories: 140
- Protein: 4g
- Carbohydrates: 12g
- Dietary Fiber: 4g
- Sugars: 2g
- Fat: 10g
- Saturated Fat: 1.5g
- Sodium: 30mg

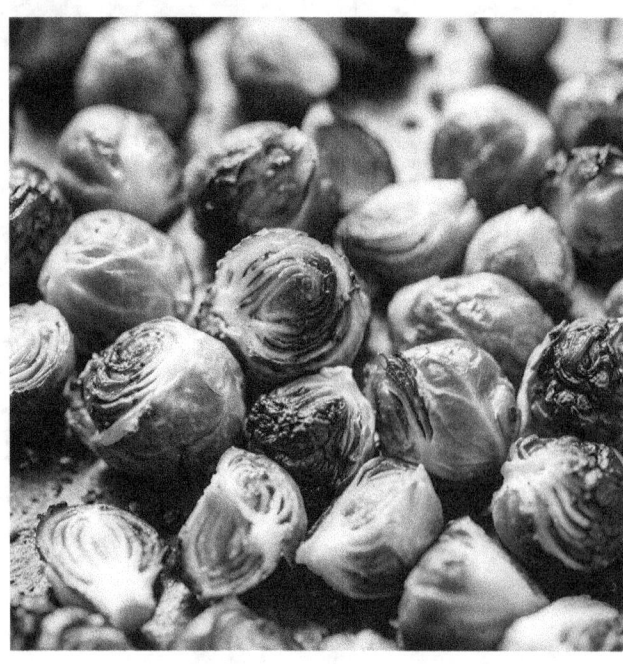

2. Kale and Quinoa Salad

Serves: 4
Cooking Time: 20 minutes
Ingredients:

- 1 cup quinoa, rinsed
- 2 cups water
- 4 cups kale, chopped
- 1 cup cherry tomatoes, halved
- 1/2 cup diced cucumber
- 1/4 cup diced red onion
- 1/4 cup crumbled feta cheese
- 3 tablespoons olive oil
- 2 tablespoons lemon juice
- 1/4 teaspoon garlic powder
- 1/4 teaspoon dried oregano

Instructions:

1. In a medium saucepan, bring water to a boil. Add quinoa, reduce heat to low, and simmer for about 15 minutes, or until the quinoa is tender and the water is absorbed. Let cool slightly.
2. In a large bowl, combine the cooked quinoa, chopped kale, cherry tomatoes, cucumber, red onion, and crumbled feta cheese.
3. In a small bowl, whisk together the olive oil, lemon juice, garlic powder, and dried oregano.
4. Pour the dressing over the salad and toss to combine.
5. Serve immediately or refrigerate for up to 2 days.

Nutrition Information (per serving):

- Calories: 220
- Protein: 7g
- Carbohydrates: 25g
- Dietary Fiber: 5g
- Sugars: 3g
- Fat: 10g
- Saturated Fat: 2.5g
- Sodium: 160mg

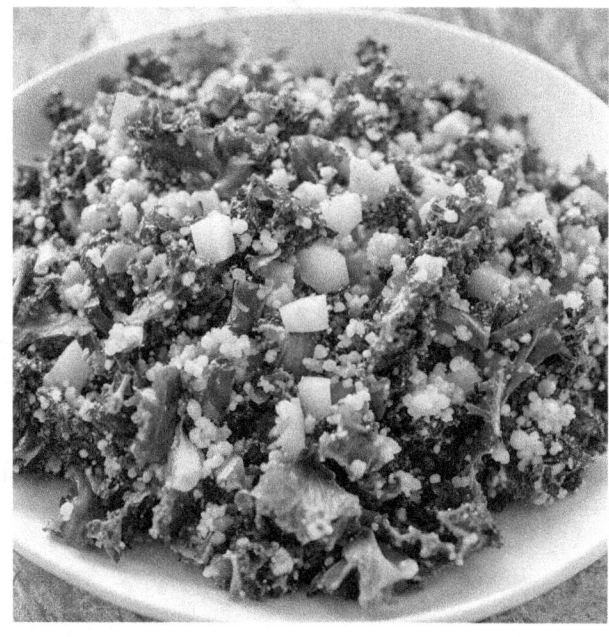

3. Zucchini Noodles with Pesto

Serves: 4

Cooking Time: 15 minutes

Ingredients:
- 4 medium zucchinis, spiralized
- 1 cup fresh basil leaves
- 1/4 cup pine nuts
- 1/4 cup grated Parmesan cheese
- 2 cloves garlic
- 1/2 cup olive oil
- 1 tablespoon lemon juice

Instructions:
1. In a food processor, combine basil leaves, pine nuts, Parmesan cheese, and garlic. Pulse until finely chopped.
2. With the processor running, slowly add the olive oil and lemon juice until the pesto is smooth.
3. In a large skillet, heat a small amount of olive oil over medium heat. Add the spiralized zucchini and sauté for 2-3 minutes, or until slightly tender.
4. Remove from heat and toss the zucchini noodles with the prepared pesto.
5. Serve immediately.

Nutrition Information (per serving):
- Calories: 240
- Protein: 5g
- Carbohydrates: 8g
- Dietary Fiber: 2g
- Sugars: 5g
- Fat: 22g
- Saturated Fat: 3.5g
- Sodium: 90mg

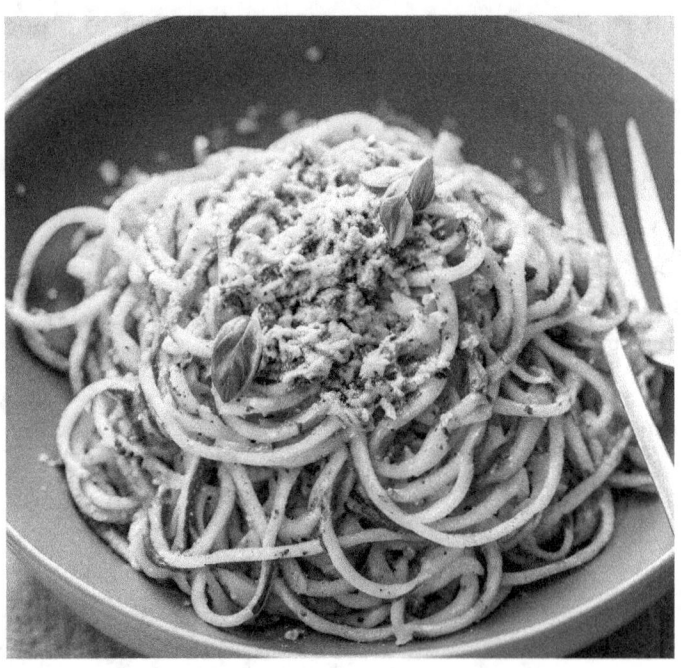

4. Butternut Squash Risotto

Serves: 4
Cooking Time: 40 minutes
Ingredients:
- 1 cup Arborio rice
- 4 cups vegetable broth, kept warm
- 2 cups butternut squash, peeled and diced
- 1 small onion, finely chopped
- 2 cloves garlic, minced
- 1/2 cup dry white wine (optional)
- 3 tablespoons olive oil
- 1/4 cup grated Parmesan cheese
- 1 tablespoon fresh thyme leaves

Instructions:
1. In a large saucepan, heat 2 tablespoons of olive oil over medium heat. Add the onion and garlic, and cook until softened, about 5 minutes.
2. Add the diced butternut squash and cook for another 5 minutes, until slightly tender.
3. Stir in the Arborio rice and cook for 1-2 minutes until the rice is lightly toasted.
4. Pour in the white wine (if using) and cook until mostly evaporated, about 2-3 minutes.
5. Begin adding the warm vegetable broth, one ladle at a time, stirring frequently. Allow the liquid to be absorbed before adding more. Continue this process for about 20 minutes, or until the rice is creamy and cooked through.
6. Stir in the remaining tablespoon of olive oil, grated Parmesan cheese, and fresh thyme leaves.
7. Remove from heat and let sit for a few minutes before serving.

Nutrition Information (per serving):
- Calories: 310
- Protein: 8g
- Carbohydrates: 45g
- Dietary Fiber: 4g
- Sugars: 4g
- Fat: 10g
- Saturated Fat: 2.5g
- Sodium: 480mg

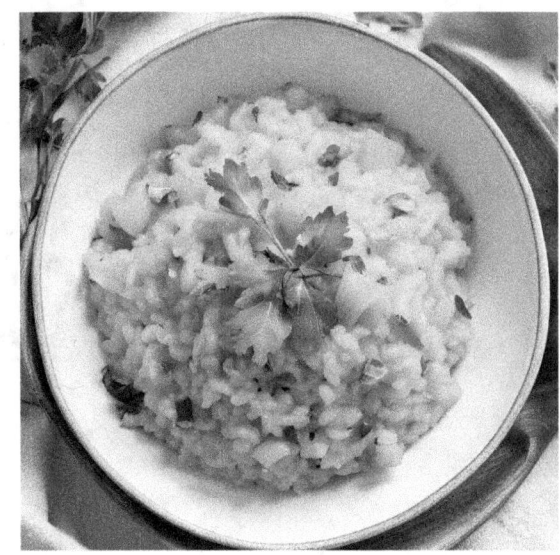

5. Spinach and Feta Stuffed Mushrooms

Serves: 4
Cooking Time: 30 minutes
Ingredients:
- 12 large button mushrooms, stems removed
- 1 tablespoon olive oil
- 1 small onion, finely chopped
- 2 cloves garlic, minced
- 2 cups fresh spinach, chopped
- 1/4 cup crumbled feta cheese
- 1/4 teaspoon dried oregano
- 1 tablespoon lemon juice

Instructions:
1. Preheat the oven to 375°F (190°C). Line a baking sheet with parchment paper.
2. In a skillet, heat olive oil over medium heat. Add the chopped onion and garlic, and cook until softened, about 5 minutes.
3. Add the chopped spinach to the skillet and cook until wilted, about 2-3 minutes. Remove from heat and let cool slightly.
4. In a bowl, combine the cooked spinach mixture, crumbled feta cheese, dried oregano, and lemon juice.
5. Stuff each mushroom cap with the spinach and feta mixture and place them on the prepared baking sheet.
6. Bake in the preheated oven for 15-20 minutes, or until the mushrooms are tender.
7. Serve warm.

Nutrition Information (per serving):
- Calories: 110
- Protein: 4g
- Carbohydrates: 8g
- Dietary Fiber: 2g
- Sugars: 2g
- Fat: 7g
- Saturated Fat: 2g
- Sodium: 150mg

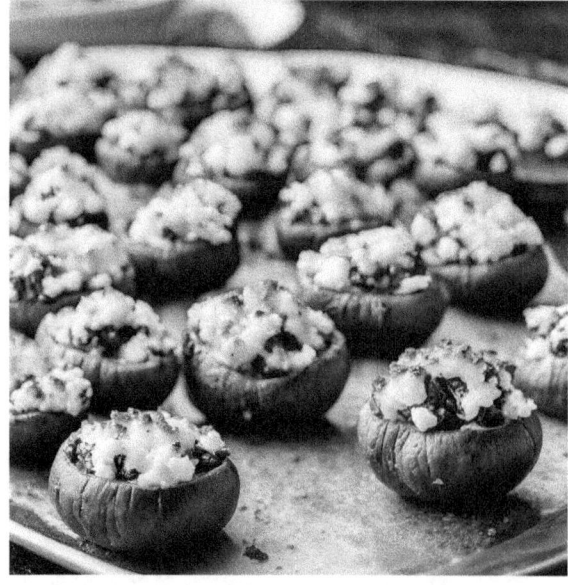

6. Grilled Eggplant with Tomato and Basil

Serves: 4
Cooking Time: 20 minutes
Ingredients:
- 2 medium eggplants, sliced into 1/2-inch rounds
- 3 tablespoons olive oil
- 2 cloves garlic, minced
- 1 cup cherry tomatoes, halved
- 1/4 cup fresh basil leaves, chopped
- 1 tablespoon balsamic vinegar

Instructions:
1. Preheat the grill to medium-high heat.
2. In a bowl, combine olive oil and minced garlic. Brush both sides of the eggplant slices with the garlic oil mixture.
3. Grill the eggplant slices for about 5 minutes on each side, or until tender and grill marks appear.
4. In a separate bowl, combine the cherry tomatoes, fresh basil, and balsamic vinegar.
5. Arrange the grilled eggplant slices on a serving platter and top with the tomato and basil mixture.
6. Serve immediately.

Nutrition Information (per serving):
- Calories: 130
- Protein: 2g
- Carbohydrates: 10g
- Dietary Fiber: 4g
- Sugars: 5g
- Fat: 9g
- Saturated Fat: 1.5g
- Sodium: 10mg

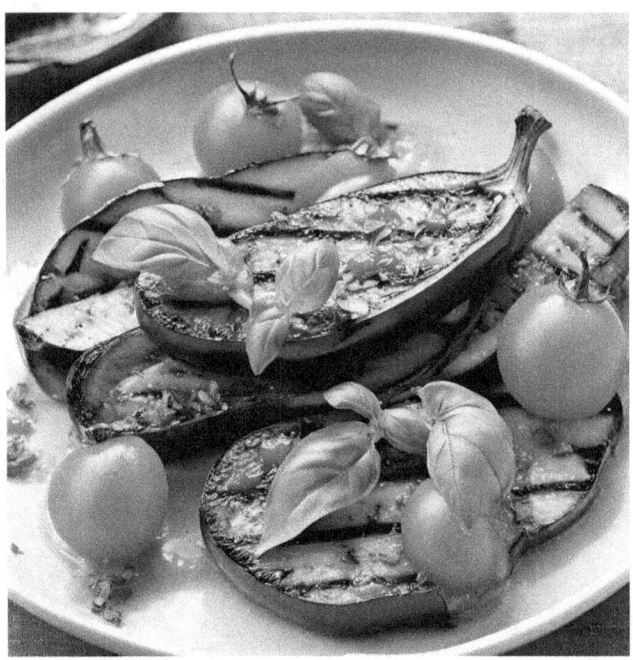

7. Green Bean Almondine

Serves: 4
Cooking Time: 15 minutes
Ingredients:

- 1 pound fresh green beans, trimmed
- 2 tablespoons olive oil
- 2 cloves garlic, minced
- 1/4 cup sliced almonds
- 1 tablespoon lemon juice

Instructions:

1. Bring a large pot of water to a boil. Add the green beans and cook for 3-4 minutes, or until tender-crisp. Drain and set aside.
2. In a large skillet, heat olive oil over medium heat. Add the minced garlic and sliced almonds, and cook until the almonds are lightly toasted, about 2-3 minutes.
3. Add the cooked green beans to the skillet and toss to coat in the garlic and almond mixture.
4. Remove from heat and drizzle with lemon juice.
5. Serve warm.

Nutrition Information (per serving):

- Calories: 120
- Protein: 3g
- Carbohydrates: 10g
- Dietary Fiber: 4g
- Sugars: 2g
- Fat: 8g
- Saturated Fat: 1g
- Sodium: 5mg

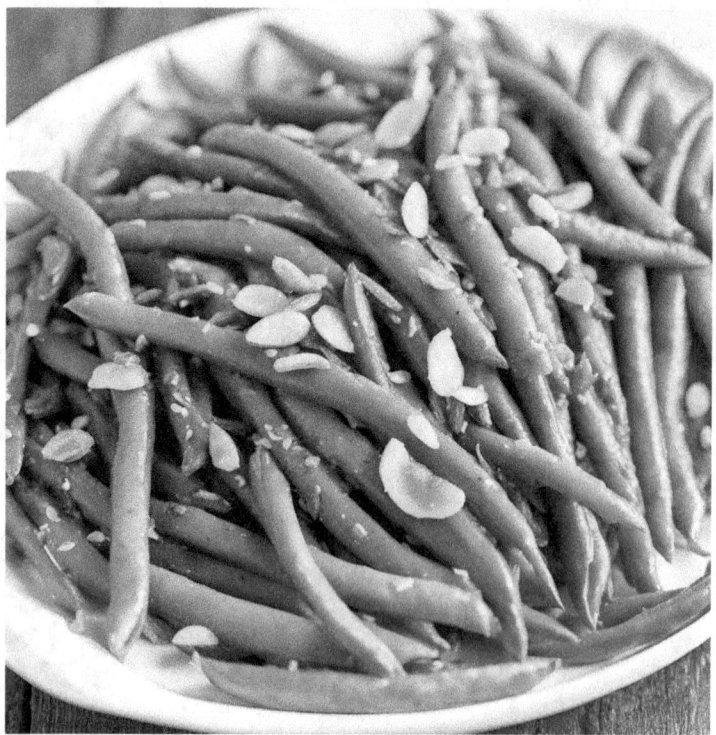

8. Roasted Turnips with Parsley

Serves: 4
Cooking Time: 30 minutes
Ingredients:
- 1 1/2 pounds turnips, peeled and cut into 1-inch pieces
- 3 tablespoons olive oil
- 2 cloves garlic, minced
- 1/4 cup fresh parsley, chopped
- 1 tablespoon lemon juice
- 1/4 teaspoon dried thyme

Instructions:
1. Preheat the oven to 400°F (200°C). Line a baking sheet with parchment paper.
2. In a large bowl, toss the turnip pieces with olive oil, minced garlic, and dried thyme until evenly coated.
3. Spread the turnips in a single layer on the prepared baking sheet.
4. Roast in the preheated oven for 25-30 minutes, or until the turnips are tender and golden brown, stirring halfway through.
5. Remove from the oven and toss with chopped parsley and lemon juice.
6. Serve warm.

Nutrition Information (per serving):
- Calories: 130
- Protein: 2g
- Carbohydrates: 12g
- Dietary Fiber: 4g
- Sugars: 5g
- Fat: 9g
- Saturated Fat: 1.5g
- Sodium: 20mg

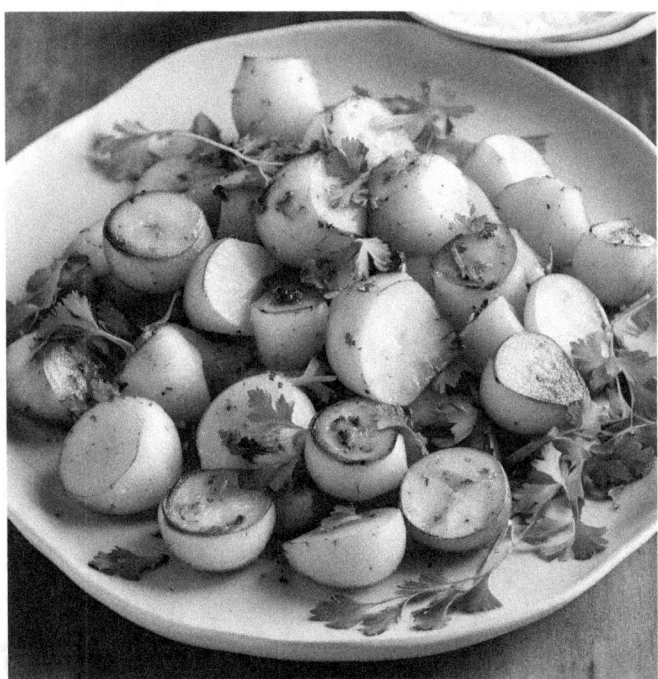

9. Stir-fried Bok Choy

Serves: 4
Cooking Time: 10 minutes
Ingredients:
- 1 1/2 pounds baby bok choy, halved lengthwise
- 2 tablespoons olive oil
- 3 cloves garlic, minced
- 1 tablespoon ginger, minced
- 2 tablespoons low-sodium soy sauce
- 1 tablespoon rice vinegar

Instructions:
1. Heat olive oil in a large skillet or wok over medium-high heat.
2. Add the minced garlic and ginger, and stir-fry for about 1 minute, until fragrant.
3. Add the bok choy and stir-fry for 3-4 minutes, until the greens are wilted and the stalks are tender-crisp.
4. Add the soy sauce and rice vinegar, and stir to combine.
5. Remove from heat and serve immediately.

Nutrition Information (per serving):
- Calories: 80
- Protein: 2g
- Carbohydrates: 8g
- Dietary Fiber: 2g
- Sugars: 2g
- Fat: 6g
- Saturated Fat: 1g
- Sodium: 300mg

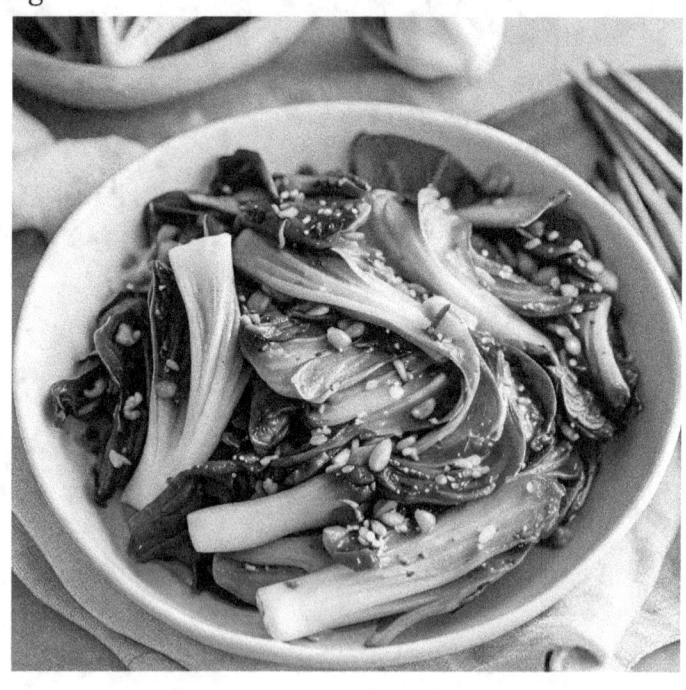

10. Vegetarian Chili

Serves: 6
Cooking Time: 45 minutes
Ingredients:

- 1 tablespoon olive oil
- 1 large onion, diced
- 3 cloves garlic, minced
- 1 red bell pepper, diced
- 1 yellow bell pepper, diced
- 2 carrots, peeled and chopped
- 1 zucchini, diced
- 1 cup corn kernels (fresh or frozen)
- 2 cans (15 oz each) black beans, rinsed and drained
- 2 cans (15 oz each) kidney beans, rinsed and drained
- 1 can (28 oz) diced tomatoes
- 2 cups vegetable broth
- 2 tablespoons chili powder
- 1 tablespoon ground cumin
- 1 teaspoon smoked paprika
- 1 teaspoon dried oregano
- 1 tablespoon apple cider vinegar

Instructions:

1. In a large pot, heat olive oil over medium heat. Add the diced onion and garlic, cooking until softened, about 5 minutes.
2. Add the red and yellow bell peppers, carrots, and zucchini to the pot. Cook for another 5-7 minutes, until the vegetables start to soften.
3. Stir in the corn kernels, black beans, kidney beans, diced tomatoes, vegetable broth, chili powder, ground cumin, smoked paprika, and dried oregano.
4. Bring the mixture to a boil, then reduce heat and simmer for 25-30 minutes, stirring occasionally.
5. Stir in the apple cider vinegar and cook for another 2 minutes.
6. Serve warm.

Nutrition Information (per serving):

- Calories: 280
- Protein: 12g
- Carbohydrates: 45g
- Dietary Fiber: 15g
- Sugars: 10g
- Fat: 6g
- Saturated Fat: 1g
- Sodium: 450mg

11. Asparagus Lemon Pasta

Serves: 4
Cooking Time: 20 minutes
Ingredients:
- 8 oz whole wheat pasta
- 1 tablespoon olive oil
- 1 bunch asparagus, trimmed and cut into 1-inch pieces
- 3 cloves garlic, minced
- 1/4 cup grated Parmesan cheese
- 1 tablespoon lemon zest
- 2 tablespoons lemon juice
- 1/4 cup chopped fresh parsley

Instructions:
1. Cook the pasta according to the package instructions. Drain and set aside.
2. In a large skillet, heat olive oil over medium heat. Add the asparagus and cook for 5-7 minutes, until tender.
3. Add the minced garlic to the skillet and cook for another 1-2 minutes, until fragrant.
4. Add the cooked pasta to the skillet, tossing to combine.
5. Remove from heat and stir in the grated Parmesan cheese, lemon zest, lemon juice, and chopped parsley.
6. Serve warm.

Nutrition Information (per serving):
- Calories: 300
- Protein: 10g
- Carbohydrates: 50g
- Dietary Fiber: 8g
- Sugars: 4g
- Fat: 8g
- Saturated Fat: 2g
- Sodium: 180mg

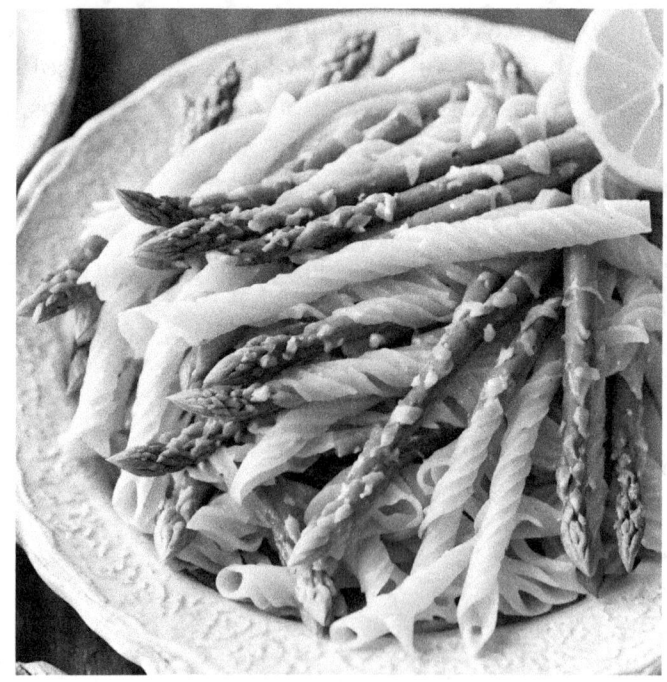

12. Cabbage Slaw with Honey Lime Dressing
Serves: 4
Cooking Time: 15 minutes
Ingredients:
- 4 cups shredded cabbage (green or purple)
- 1 cup shredded carrots
- 1/4 cup chopped fresh cilantro
- 1/4 cup olive oil
- 3 tablespoons lime juice
- 1 tablespoon honey
- 1/4 teaspoon cumin
- 1/4 teaspoon garlic powder

Instructions:
1. In a large bowl, combine the shredded cabbage, shredded carrots, and chopped cilantro.
2. In a small bowl, whisk together the olive oil, lime juice, honey, cumin, and garlic powder.
3. Pour the dressing over the cabbage mixture and toss to combine.
4. Serve immediately or refrigerate for up to 2 days.

Nutrition Information (per serving):
- Calories: 180
- Protein: 2g
- Carbohydrates: 15g
- Dietary Fiber: 4g
- Sugars: 8g
- Fat: 14g
- Saturated Fat: 2g
- Sodium: 10mg

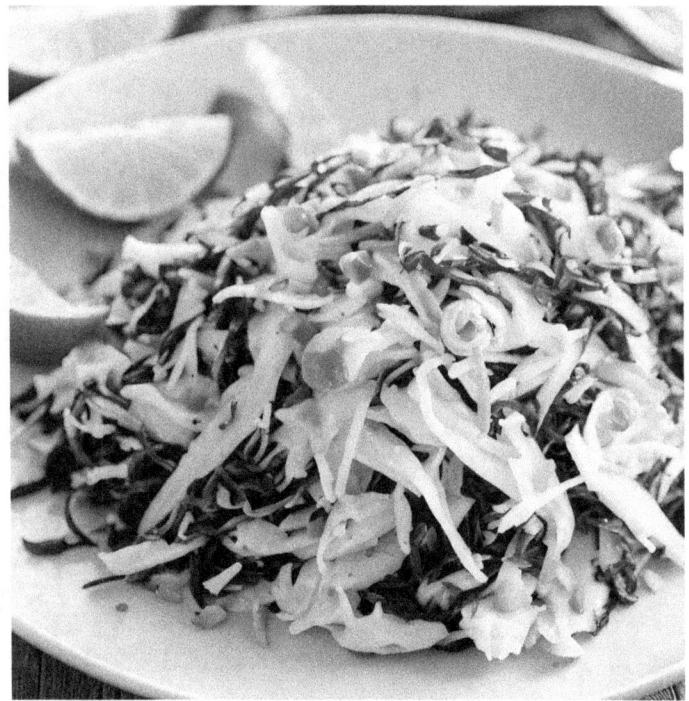

13. Sautéed Swiss Chard with Pine Nuts

Serves: 4

Cooking Time: 15 minutes

Ingredients:
- 1 bunch Swiss chard, stems removed and leaves chopped
- 2 tablespoons olive oil
- 3 cloves garlic, minced
- 1/4 cup pine nuts
- 1 tablespoon lemon juice
- 1/4 teaspoon crushed red pepper flakes

Instructions:
1. In a large skillet, heat olive oil over medium heat. Add the minced garlic and cook for 1-2 minutes, until fragrant.
2. Add the chopped Swiss chard to the skillet and cook for 5-7 minutes, until wilted.
3. Stir in the pine nuts and cook for another 2 minutes, until lightly toasted.
4. Remove from heat and stir in the lemon juice and crushed red pepper flakes.
5. Serve warm.

Nutrition Information (per serving):
- Calories: 140
- Protein: 2g
- Carbohydrates: 6g
- Dietary Fiber: 2g
- Sugars: 1g
- Fat: 12g
- Saturated Fat: 1.5g
- Sodium: 30mg

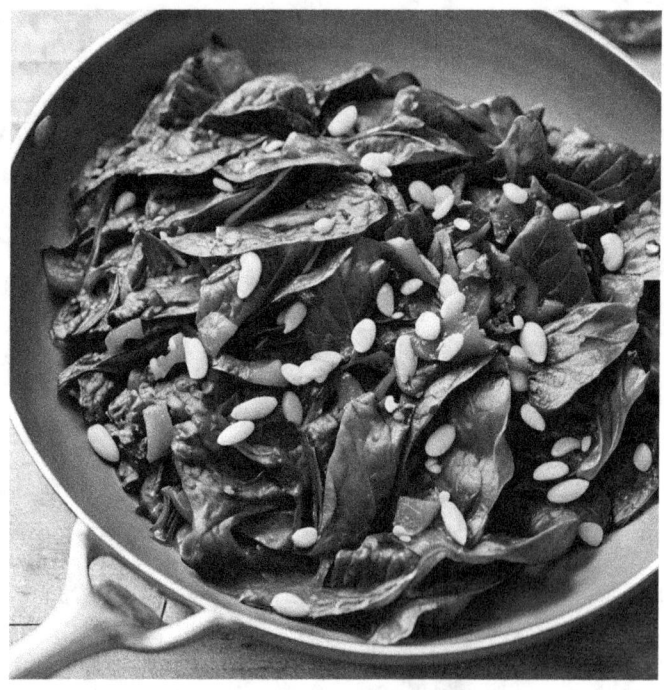

14. Spaghetti Squash Primavera

Serves: 4
Cooking Time: 45 minutes
Ingredients:

- 1 large spaghetti squash
- 2 tablespoons olive oil, divided
- 1 small onion, diced
- 2 cloves garlic, minced
- 1 red bell pepper, diced
- 1 zucchini, diced
- 1 cup cherry tomatoes, halved
- 1 cup fresh spinach, chopped
- 1/4 teaspoon dried oregano
- 1/4 teaspoon dried basil
- 1/4 cup grated Parmesan cheese
- 1 tablespoon lemon juice

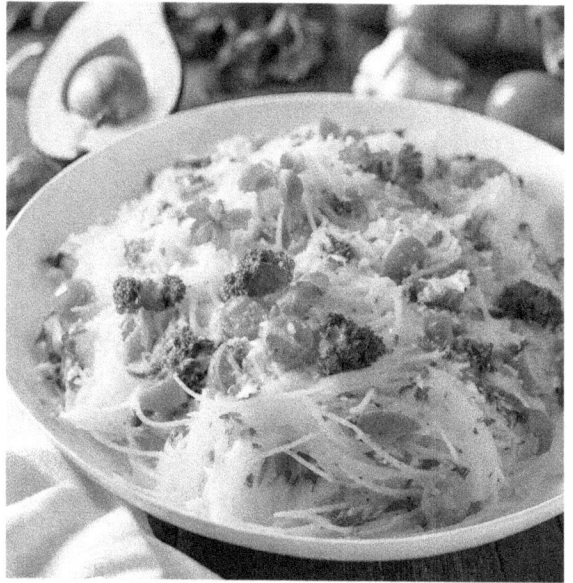

Instructions:

1. Preheat the oven to 400°F (200°C). Line a baking sheet with parchment paper.
2. Cut the spaghetti squash in half lengthwise and scoop out the seeds. Brush the cut sides with 1 tablespoon of olive oil and place them cut side down on the prepared baking sheet.
3. Roast the squash in the preheated oven for 35-40 minutes, or until the flesh is tender and can be easily scraped into strands with a fork.
4. While the squash is roasting, heat the remaining 1 tablespoon of olive oil in a large skillet over medium heat. Add the diced onion and cook until softened, about 5 minutes.
5. Add the garlic, red bell pepper, and zucchini to the skillet. Cook for another 5-7 minutes, until the vegetables are tender.
6. Stir in the cherry tomatoes, spinach, oregano, and basil. Cook until the spinach is wilted, about 2-3 minutes.
7. Remove the spaghetti squash from the oven and use a fork to scrape the flesh into spaghetti-like strands.
8. Add the spaghetti squash strands to the skillet with the vegetables and toss to combine.
9. Remove from heat and stir in the grated Parmesan cheese and lemon juice.
10. Serve warm.

Nutrition Information (per serving):

- Calories: 180 Protein: 5g Carbohydrates: 20g Dietary Fiber: 5g
- Sugars: 8g Fat: 10g Saturated Fat: 2g
- Sodium: 80mg

15. Roasted Radishes with Rosemary

Serves: 4
Cooking Time: 25 minutes
Ingredients:
- 2 bunches radishes, trimmed and halved
- 2 tablespoons olive oil
- 1 tablespoon fresh rosemary, chopped
- 1 tablespoon lemon juice

Instructions:
1. Preheat the oven to 425°F (220°C). Line a baking sheet with parchment paper.
2. In a large bowl, toss the halved radishes with olive oil and chopped rosemary until evenly coated.
3. Spread the radishes in a single layer on the prepared baking sheet.
4. Roast in the preheated oven for 20-25 minutes, or until the radishes are tender and golden brown, stirring halfway through.
5. Remove from the oven and drizzle with lemon juice before serving.
6. Serve warm.

Nutrition Information (per serving):
- Calories: 80
- Protein: 1g
- Carbohydrates: 6g
- Dietary Fiber: 2g
- Sugars: 3g
- Fat: 7g
- Saturated Fat: 1g
- Sodium: 10mg

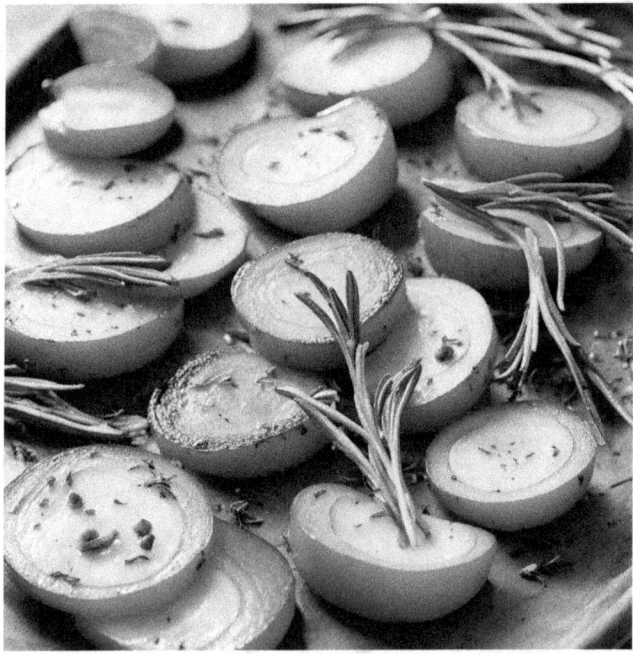

16. Eggplant Caponata

Serves: 4
Cooking Time: 40 minutes
Ingredients:

- 2 medium eggplants, diced
- 1/4 cup olive oil
- 1 small onion, diced
- 2 cloves garlic, minced
- 1 red bell pepper, diced
- 1 can (15 oz) diced tomatoes
- 1/4 cup green olives, sliced
- 2 tablespoons capers, rinsed
- 2 tablespoons red wine vinegar
- 1 tablespoon honey or maple syrup
- 1/4 teaspoon dried oregano
- 1/4 teaspoon crushed red pepper flakes (optional)
- 1/4 cup chopped fresh parsley

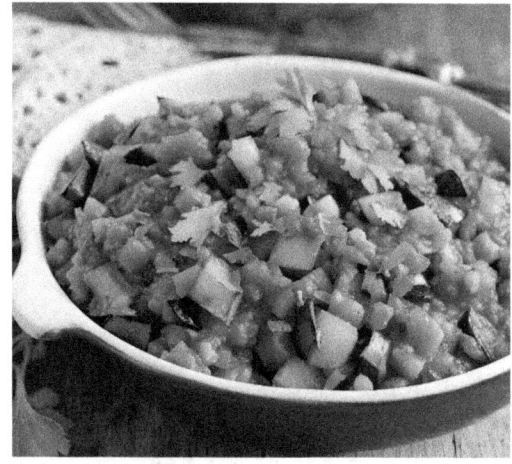

Instructions:

1. In a large skillet, heat the olive oil over medium heat. Add the diced eggplant and cook, stirring occasionally, until the eggplant is softened and golden brown, about 10 minutes.
2. Add the diced onion, garlic, and red bell pepper to the skillet. Cook for another 5-7 minutes, until the vegetables are tender.
3. Stir in the diced tomatoes (with their juices), green olives, capers, red wine vinegar, honey or maple syrup, oregano, and crushed red pepper flakes if using.
4. Bring the mixture to a simmer and cook for 15-20 minutes, stirring occasionally, until the flavors are well combined and the caponata is thickened.
5. Remove from heat and stir in the chopped fresh parsley.
6. Serve warm or at room temperature.

Nutrition Information (per serving):

- Calories: 200
- Protein: 2g
- Carbohydrates: 18g
- Dietary Fiber: 6g
- Sugars: 10g
- Fat: 14g
- Saturated Fat: 2g
- Sodium: 320mg

Poultry Recipes

1. Grilled Chicken Salad
Serves: 4
Cooking Time: 30 minutes
Ingredients:
- 4 boneless, skinless chicken breasts
- 2 tablespoons olive oil
- 1 tablespoon lemon juice
- 1 teaspoon garlic powder
- 1 teaspoon dried oregano
- 8 cups mixed greens (such as spinach, arugula, and lettuce)
- 1 cup cherry tomatoes, halved
- 1 cucumber, sliced
- 1/4 cup red onion, thinly sliced
- 1/4 cup crumbled feta cheese
- 2 tablespoons balsamic vinegar

Instructions:
1. Preheat the grill to medium-high heat.
2. In a small bowl, mix the olive oil, lemon juice, garlic powder, and dried oregano. Brush the mixture over the chicken breasts.
3. Grill the chicken breasts for 6-8 minutes per side, or until fully cooked and the internal temperature reaches 165°F (75°C). Remove from grill and let rest for 5 minutes before slicing.
4. In a large bowl, combine the mixed greens, cherry tomatoes, cucumber, red onion, and crumbled feta cheese.
5. Top the salad with sliced grilled chicken.
6. Drizzle with balsamic vinegar before serving.

Nutrition Information (per serving):
- Calories: 320
- Protein: 30g
- Carbohydrates: 10g
- Dietary Fiber: 4g
- Sugars: 5g
- Fat: 18g
- Saturated Fat: 4g
- Sodium: 220mg

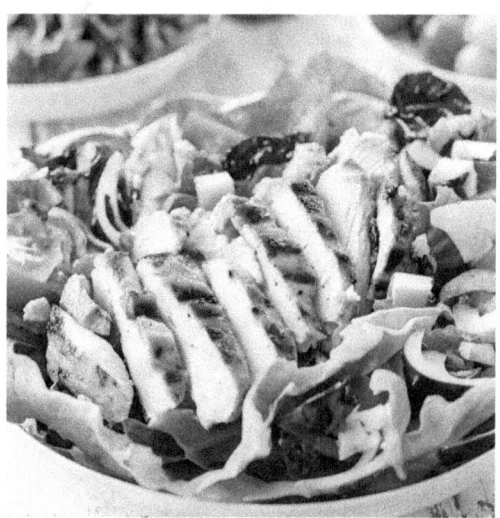

2. Turkey Chili

Serves: 6
Cooking Time: 1 hour
Ingredients:
- 1 tablespoon olive oil
- 1 large onion, diced
- 3 cloves garlic, minced
- 1 red bell pepper, diced
- 1 green bell pepper, diced
- 1 pound ground turkey
- 1 can (15 oz) black beans, rinsed and drained
- 1 can (15 oz) kidney beans, rinsed and drained
- 1 can (28 oz) diced tomatoes
- 2 cups vegetable broth
- 2 tablespoons chili powder
- 1 tablespoon ground cumin
- 1 teaspoon smoked paprika
- 1 teaspoon dried oregano
- 1 tablespoon apple cider vinegar

Instructions:
1. In a large pot, heat olive oil over medium heat. Add the diced onion and garlic, and cook until softened, about 5 minutes.
2. Add the red and green bell peppers, and cook for another 5 minutes.
3. Add the ground turkey to the pot, breaking it up with a spoon, and cook until browned, about 8-10 minutes.
4. Stir in the black beans, kidney beans, diced tomatoes, vegetable broth, chili powder, ground cumin, smoked paprika, and dried oregano.
5. Bring the mixture to a boil, then reduce heat and simmer for 30-40 minutes, stirring occasionally.
6. Stir in the apple cider vinegar and cook for another 2 minutes.
7. Serve warm.

Nutrition Information (per serving):
- Calories: 280
- Protein: 20g
- Carbohydrates: 35g
- Dietary Fiber: 12g
- Sugars: 8g
- Fat: 8g
- Saturated Fat: 1.5g
- Sodium: 320mg

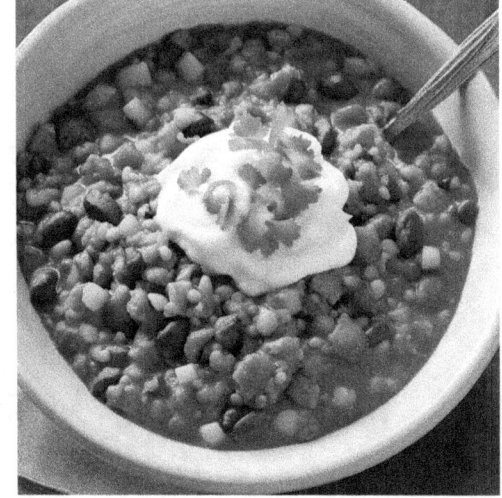

3. Chicken Stir-fry

Serves: 4
Cooking Time: 20 minutes
Ingredients:
- 2 tablespoons olive oil
- 1 pound boneless, skinless chicken breast, thinly sliced
- 2 cloves garlic, minced
- 1 tablespoon ginger, minced
- 1 red bell pepper, sliced
- 1 yellow bell pepper, sliced
- 1 cup broccoli florets
- 1 cup snap peas
- 3 tablespoons low-sodium soy sauce
- 1 tablespoon rice vinegar
- 1 tablespoon honey or maple syrup (optional)
- 1/4 teaspoon crushed red pepper flakes (optional)

Instructions:
1. Heat 1 tablespoon of olive oil in a large skillet or wok over medium-high heat.
2. Add the sliced chicken breast and cook until no longer pink, about 5-7 minutes. Remove from skillet and set aside.
3. Add the remaining 1 tablespoon of olive oil to the skillet. Add the garlic and ginger, and cook for 1-2 minutes until fragrant.
4. Add the red bell pepper, yellow bell pepper, broccoli florets, and snap peas. Stir-fry for 5-7 minutes, or until the vegetables are tender-crisp.
5. Return the cooked chicken to the skillet.
6. In a small bowl, mix the soy sauce, rice vinegar, honey or maple syrup (if using), and crushed red pepper flakes (if using). Pour the sauce over the chicken and vegetables, tossing to combine.
7. Cook for another 2-3 minutes, until the sauce is heated through.
8. Serve immediately.

Nutrition Information (per serving):
- Calories: 290
- Protein: 28g
- Carbohydrates: 15g
- Dietary Fiber: 4g
- Sugars: 7g
- Fat: 12g
- Saturated Fat: 2g
- Sodium: 480mg

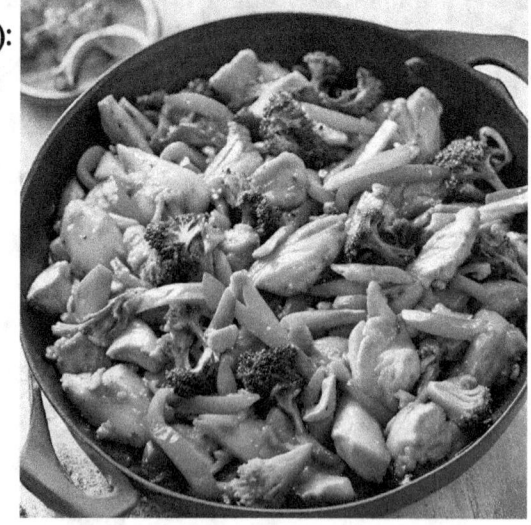

4. Roasted Turkey Breast

Serves: 4
Cooking Time: 1 hour 15 minutes
Ingredients:
- 1 (2-pound) boneless turkey breast, skin removed
- 2 tablespoons olive oil
- 2 cloves garlic, minced
- 1 teaspoon dried thyme
- 1 teaspoon dried rosemary
- 1 tablespoon lemon juice

Instructions:
1. Preheat the oven to 375°F (190°C).
2. In a small bowl, mix together olive oil, minced garlic, dried thyme, dried rosemary, and lemon juice.
3. Rub the mixture all over the turkey breast.
4. Place the turkey breast in a roasting pan.
5. Roast in the preheated oven for 60-75 minutes, or until the internal temperature reaches 165°F (75°C).
6. Let the turkey breast rest for 10 minutes before slicing.
7. Serve warm.

Nutrition Information (per serving):
- Calories: 260
- Protein: 38g
- Carbohydrates: 1g
- Dietary Fiber: 0g
- Sugars: 0g
- Fat: 12g
- Saturated Fat: 2g
- Sodium: 80mg

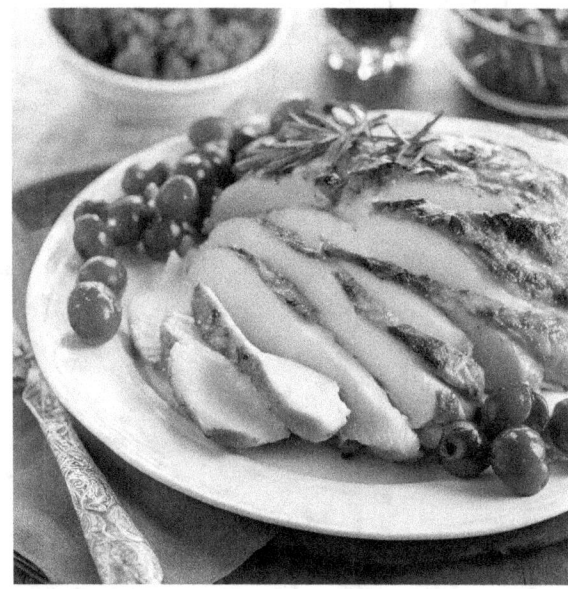

5. Chicken Zoodle Soup
Serves: 4
Cooking Time: 30 minutes
Ingredients:
- 1 tablespoon olive oil
- 1 onion, diced
- 3 cloves garlic, minced
- 2 carrots, diced
- 2 celery stalks, diced
- 1 teaspoon dried thyme
- 1 teaspoon dried basil
- 6 cups low-sodium chicken broth
- 2 cups cooked shredded chicken breast
- 2 medium zucchinis, spiralized into zoodles
- 1 tablespoon lemon juice

Instructions:
1. In a large pot, heat olive oil over medium heat. Add the diced onion and garlic, cooking until softened, about 5 minutes.
2. Add the carrots, celery, dried thyme, and dried basil. Cook for another 5 minutes, stirring occasionally.
3. Pour in the chicken broth and bring to a boil.
4. Reduce heat and simmer for 10 minutes, until the vegetables are tender.
5. Add the shredded chicken and spiralized zucchini. Cook for another 5 minutes, until the chicken is heated through and the zoodles are tender.
6. Stir in the lemon juice before serving.
7. Serve warm.

Nutrition Information (per serving):
- Calories: 180
- Protein: 20g
- Carbohydrates: 12g
- Dietary Fiber: 3g
- Sugars: 5g
- Fat: 6g
- Saturated Fat: 1g
- Sodium: 250mg

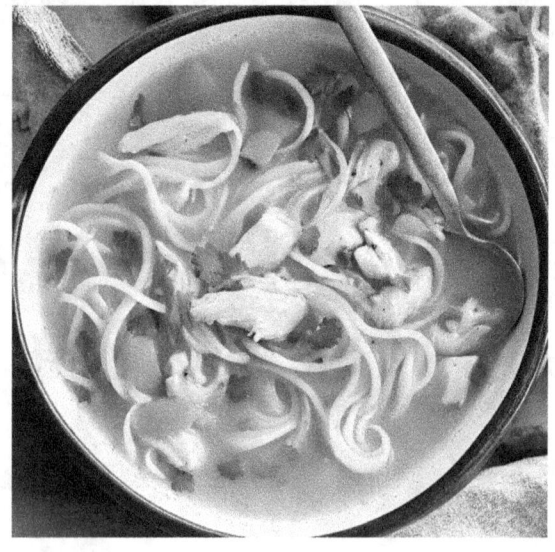

6. Baked Chicken Thighs with Dijon Mustard

Serves: 4

Cooking Time: 45 minutes

Ingredients:
- 8 bone-in, skinless chicken thighs
- 3 tablespoons Dijon mustard
- 2 tablespoons olive oil
- 2 cloves garlic, minced
- 1 teaspoon dried thyme
- 1 tablespoon lemon juice

Instructions:
1. Preheat the oven to 375°F (190°C). Line a baking dish with parchment paper.
2. In a small bowl, mix together Dijon mustard, olive oil, minced garlic, dried thyme, and lemon juice.
3. Rub the mustard mixture all over the chicken thighs.
4. Place the chicken thighs in the prepared baking dish.
5. Bake in the preheated oven for 40-45 minutes, or until the internal temperature reaches 165°F (75°C).
6. Let the chicken rest for 5 minutes before serving.
7. Serve warm.

Nutrition Information (per serving):
- Calories: 280
- Protein: 25g
- Carbohydrates: 2g
- Dietary Fiber: 0g
- Sugars: 1g
- Fat: 18g
- Saturated Fat: 4g
- Sodium: 200mg

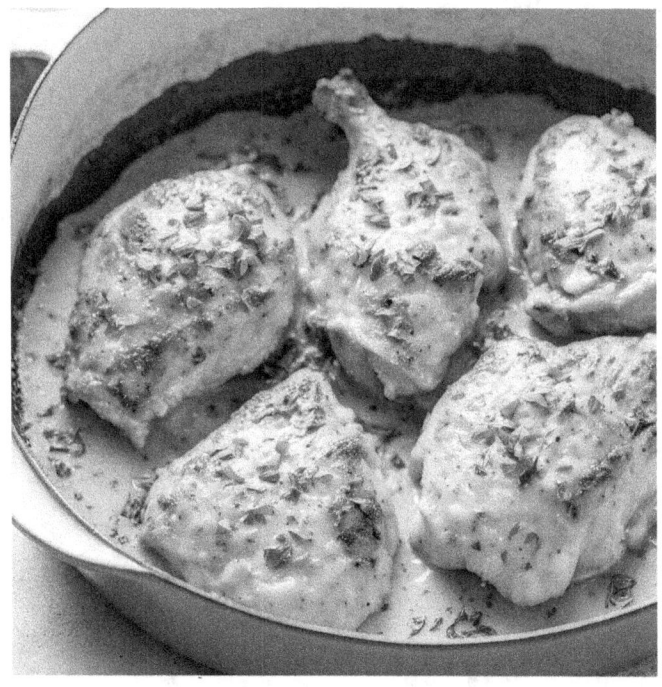

7. Turkey Meatballs in Marinara Sauce

Serves: 4
Cooking Time: 40 minutes
Ingredients:
For the Meatballs:
- 1 pound ground turkey
- 1/4 cup almond flour
- 1 egg, beaten
- 2 cloves garlic, minced
- 1 teaspoon dried oregano
- 1 teaspoon dried basil

For the Marinara Sauce:
- 1 tablespoon olive oil
- 1 onion, diced
- 2 cloves garlic, minced
- 1 can (28 oz) crushed tomatoes
- 1 teaspoon dried oregano
- 1 teaspoon dried basil
- 1 tablespoon balsamic vinegar

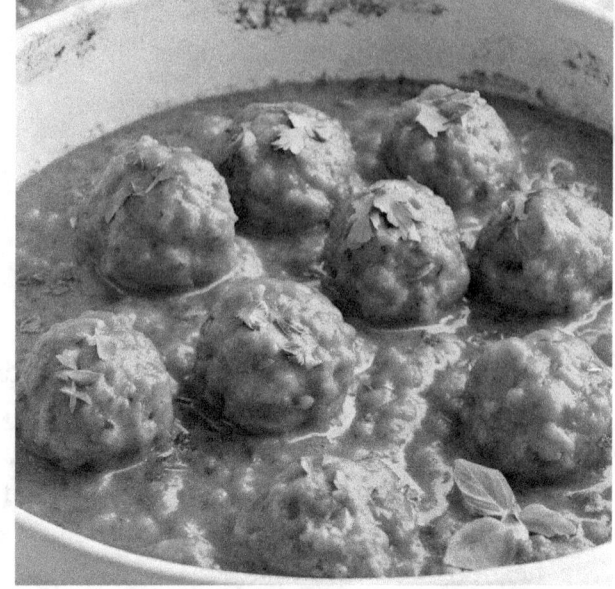

Instructions:
1. Preheat the oven to 375°F (190°C). Line a baking sheet with parchment paper.
2. In a large bowl, mix together the ground turkey, almond flour, beaten egg, minced garlic, dried oregano, and dried basil until well combined.
3. Form the mixture into meatballs and place them on the prepared baking sheet.
4. Bake in the preheated oven for 20-25 minutes, or until fully cooked.
5. While the meatballs are baking, heat olive oil in a large saucepan over medium heat. Add the diced onion and minced garlic, cooking until softened, about 5 minutes.
6. Stir in the crushed tomatoes, dried oregano, dried basil, and balsamic vinegar. Bring to a simmer and cook for 15-20 minutes, until the sauce is thickened.
7. Add the cooked meatballs to the marinara sauce and simmer for an additional 5 minutes.
8. Serve warm.

Nutrition Information (per serving):
- Calories: 300
- Protein: 25g
- Carbohydrates: 12g
- Dietary Fiber: 3g
- Sugars: 7g
- Fat: 16g
- Saturated Fat: 3g
- Sodium: 300mg

8. Chicken Stuffed Bell Peppers

Serves: 4
Cooking Time: 45 minutes

Ingredients:
- 4 large bell peppers, tops cut off and seeds removed
- 1 pound ground chicken
- 1 tablespoon olive oil
- 1 onion, diced
- 2 cloves garlic, minced
- 1 zucchini, diced
- 1 cup cooked quinoa
- 1 teaspoon dried oregano
- 1 teaspoon dried basil
- 1/2 cup marinara sauce
- 1/4 cup grated Parmesan cheese

Instructions:
1. Preheat the oven to 375°F (190°C).
2. In a large skillet, heat olive oil over medium heat. Add the diced onion and garlic, cooking until softened, about 5 minutes.
3. Add the ground chicken to the skillet and cook until browned, about 8-10 minutes.
4. Stir in the diced zucchini, cooked quinoa, dried oregano, dried basil, and marinara sauce. Cook for another 5 minutes, until the zucchini is tender.
5. Stuff each bell pepper with the chicken and quinoa mixture.
6. Place the stuffed bell peppers in a baking dish and cover with foil.
7. Bake in the preheated oven for 30 minutes.
8. Remove the foil, sprinkle grated Parmesan cheese over each pepper, and bake for an additional 5 minutes, until the cheese is melted.
9. Serve warm.

Nutrition Information (per serving):
- Calories: 350
- Protein: 30g
- Carbohydrates: 25g
- Dietary Fiber: 6g
- Sugars: 10g
- Fat: 14g
- Saturated Fat: 3g
- Sodium: 350mg

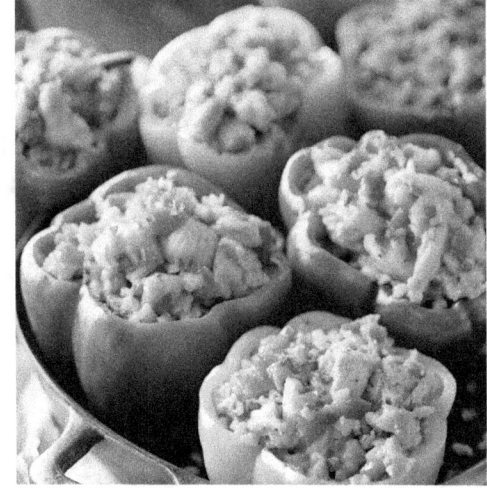

9. Herb-Roasted Turkey Legs

Serves: 4

Cooking Time: 1 hour 30 minutes

Ingredients:
- 4 turkey legs
- 3 tablespoons olive oil
- 2 cloves garlic, minced
- 1 teaspoon dried rosemary
- 1 teaspoon dried thyme
- 1 teaspoon dried sage
- 1 tablespoon lemon juice

Instructions:
1. Preheat the oven to 375°F (190°C).
2. In a small bowl, mix together olive oil, minced garlic, dried rosemary, dried thyme, dried sage, and lemon juice.
3. Rub the herb mixture all over the turkey legs.
4. Place the turkey legs in a roasting pan.
5. Roast in the preheated oven for 90 minutes, or until the internal temperature reaches 165°F (75°C).
6. Let the turkey legs rest for 10 minutes before serving.
7. Serve warm.

Nutrition Information (per serving):
- Calories: 350
- Protein: 40g
- Carbohydrates: 1g
- Dietary Fiber: 0g
- Sugars: 0g
- Fat: 20g
- Saturated Fat: 4g
- Sodium: 90mg

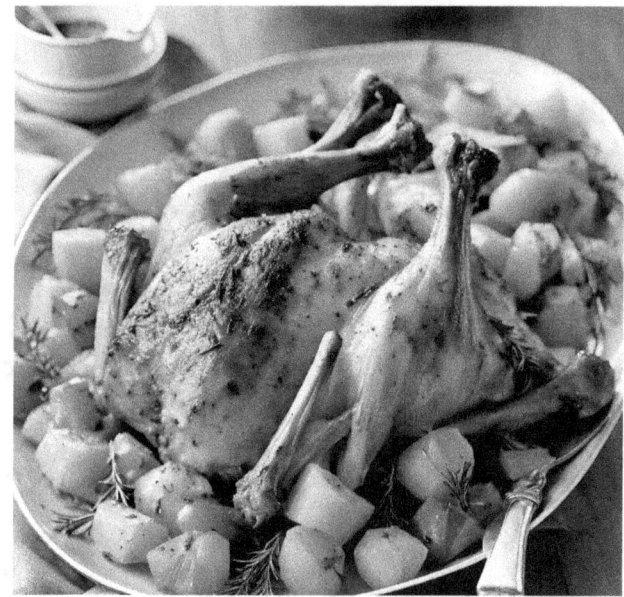

10. Chicken and Spinach Curry

Serves: 4
Cooking Time: 30 minutes
Ingredients:
- 2 tablespoons olive oil
- 1 onion, diced
- 3 cloves garlic, minced
- 1 tablespoon fresh ginger, minced
- 1 pound boneless, skinless chicken breasts, cut into bite-sized pieces
- 1 tablespoon curry powder
- 1 teaspoon ground cumin
- 1 teaspoon ground coriander
- 1 can (14 oz) coconut milk
- 4 cups fresh spinach, chopped
- 1 tablespoon lemon juice

Instructions:
1. Heat olive oil in a large skillet over medium heat. Add the diced onion, garlic, and ginger, cooking until softened, about 5 minutes.
2. Add the chicken pieces to the skillet and cook until browned, about 5-7 minutes.
3. Stir in the curry powder, ground cumin, and ground coriander, cooking for another 2 minutes.
4. Pour in the coconut milk and bring to a simmer. Cook for 10 minutes, until the chicken is fully cooked.
5. Add the chopped spinach to the skillet and cook until wilted, about 2-3 minutes.
6. Stir in the lemon juice before serving.
7. Serve warm.

Nutrition Information (per serving):
- Calories: 340
- Protein: 30g
- Carbohydrates: 8g
- Dietary Fiber: 3g
- Sugars: 2g
- Fat: 20g
- Saturated Fat: 12g
- Sodium: 180mg

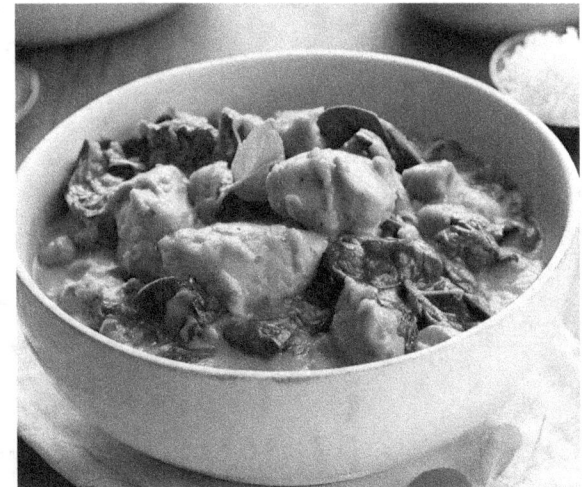

11. Turkey Lettuce Wraps

Serves: 4
Cooking Time: 20 minutes
Ingredients:
- 1 tablespoon olive oil
- 1 pound ground turkey
- 2 cloves garlic, minced
- 1 small onion, diced
- 1 carrot, grated
- 1 red bell pepper, diced
- 3 tablespoons low-sodium soy sauce
- 1 tablespoon rice vinegar
- 1 tablespoon honey or maple syrup (optional)
- 1 head butter lettuce, leaves separated
- 1/4 cup chopped fresh cilantro

Instructions:
1. Heat olive oil in a large skillet over medium heat. Add the ground turkey and cook until browned, about 8-10 minutes.
2. Add the minced garlic, diced onion, grated carrot, and red bell pepper. Cook for another 5 minutes, until the vegetables are tender.
3. Stir in the soy sauce, rice vinegar, and honey or maple syrup (if using). Cook for another 2 minutes.
4. Spoon the turkey mixture into lettuce leaves and top with chopped fresh cilantro.
5. Serve immediately.

Nutrition Information (per serving):
- Calories: 250
- Protein: 28g
- Carbohydrates: 10g
- Dietary Fiber: 2g
- Sugars: 5g
- Fat: 12g
- Saturated Fat: 2g
- Sodium: 300mg

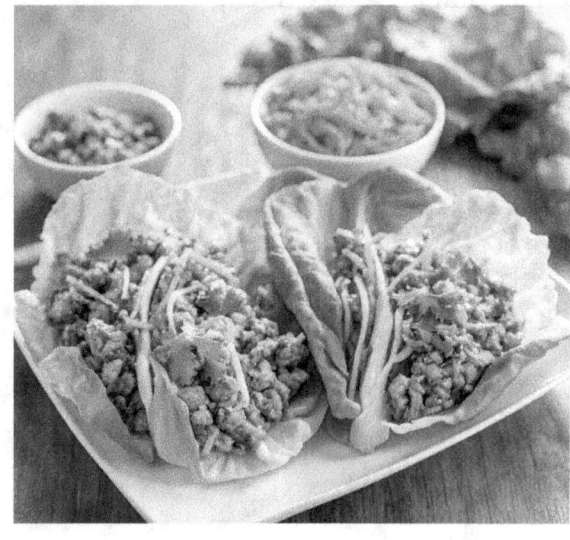

12. Chicken and Vegetable Kebabs

Serves: 4
Cooking Time: 20 minutes
Ingredients:

- 1 pound boneless, skinless chicken breasts, cut into 1-inch cubes
- 1 red bell pepper, cut into 1-inch pieces
- 1 yellow bell pepper, cut into 1-inch pieces
- 1 zucchini, sliced into 1/2-inch rounds
- 1 red onion, cut into wedges
- 3 tablespoons olive oil
- 1 tablespoon lemon juice
- 1 teaspoon dried oregano
- 1 teaspoon garlic powder

Instructions:

1. Preheat the grill to medium-high heat.
2. In a large bowl, combine olive oil, lemon juice, dried oregano, and garlic powder. Add the chicken cubes and vegetables, tossing to coat evenly.
3. Thread the chicken and vegetables onto skewers.
4. Grill the kebabs for 10-12 minutes, turning occasionally, until the chicken is fully cooked and the vegetables are tender.
5. Serve immediately.

Nutrition Information (per serving):

- Calories: 260
- Protein: 25g
- Carbohydrates: 10g
- Dietary Fiber: 3g
- Sugars: 5g
- Fat: 14g
- Saturated Fat: 2.5g
- Sodium: 100mg

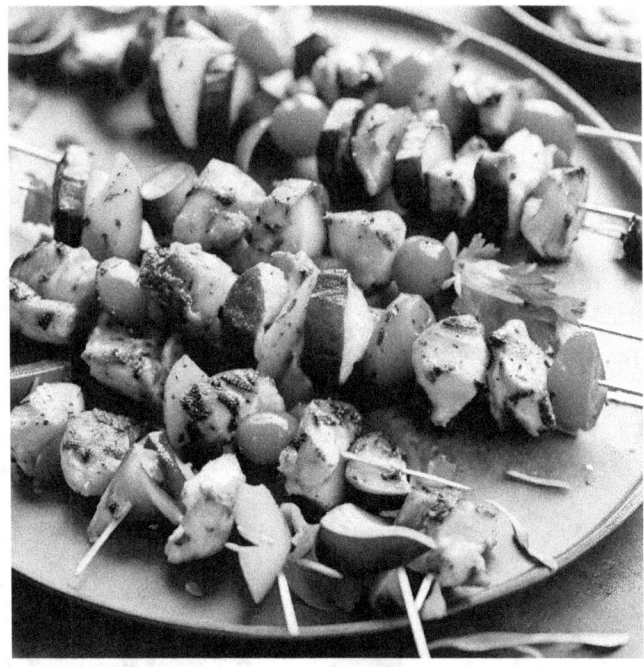

13. Buffalo Chicken Salad

Serves: 4
Cooking Time: 20 minutes

Ingredients:
- 1 pound boneless, skinless chicken breasts, cut into strips
- 3 tablespoons olive oil
- 1/4 cup hot sauce (such as Frank's RedHot)
- 1 head romaine lettuce, chopped
- 1 cup cherry tomatoes, halved
- 1/2 cup shredded carrots
- 1/4 cup diced celery
- 1/4 cup crumbled blue cheese
- 1 tablespoon lemon juice

Instructions:
1. Heat olive oil in a large skillet over medium heat. Add the chicken strips and cook until fully cooked, about 8-10 minutes.
2. Remove the skillet from heat and stir in the hot sauce, coating the chicken evenly.
3. In a large bowl, combine the chopped romaine lettuce, cherry tomatoes, shredded carrots, and diced celery.
4. Top the salad with the buffalo chicken and crumbled blue cheese.
5. Drizzle with lemon juice before serving.
6. Serve immediately.

Nutrition Information (per serving):
- Calories: 320
- Protein: 30g
- Carbohydrates: 10g
- Dietary Fiber: 4g
- Sugars: 4g
- Fat: 18g
- Saturated Fat: 5g
- Sodium: 700mg

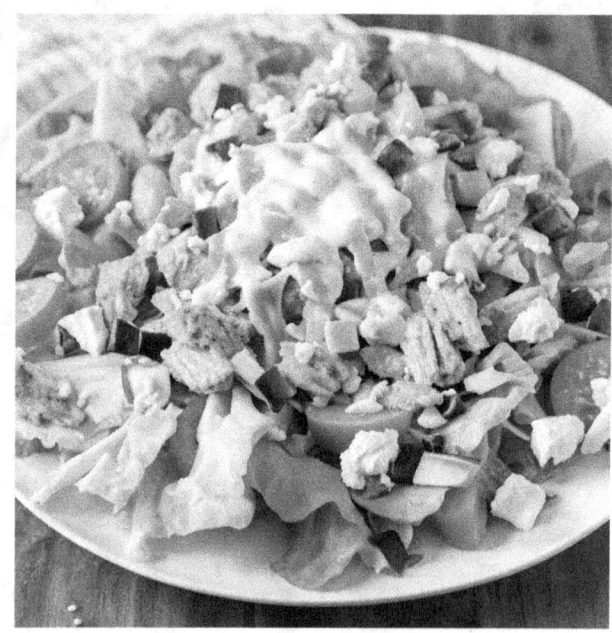

14. Turkey and Sweet Potato Hash

Serves: 4
Cooking Time: 30 minutes
Ingredients:

- 2 tablespoons olive oil
- 1 pound ground turkey
- 1 large sweet potato, peeled and diced
- 1 small onion, diced
- 1 red bell pepper, diced
- 1 teaspoon garlic powder
- 1 teaspoon dried thyme
- 1 tablespoon apple cider vinegar
- 1/4 cup chopped fresh parsley

Instructions:

1. In a large skillet, heat 1 tablespoon of olive oil over medium heat. Add the ground turkey and cook until browned, about 8-10 minutes. Remove from skillet and set aside.
2. Add the remaining 1 tablespoon of olive oil to the skillet. Add the sweet potato and cook for about 10 minutes, until tender, stirring occasionally.
3. Add the onion and red bell pepper, cooking for another 5 minutes, until softened.
4. Return the cooked turkey to the skillet and stir in the garlic powder, dried thyme, and apple cider vinegar. Cook for an additional 2-3 minutes, until everything is heated through.
5. Sprinkle with chopped fresh parsley before serving.
6. Serve warm.

Nutrition Information (per serving):

- Calories: 280
- Protein: 24g
- Carbohydrates: 20g
- Dietary Fiber: 4g
- Sugars: 6g
- Fat: 12g
- Saturated Fat: 2.5g
- Sodium: 200mg

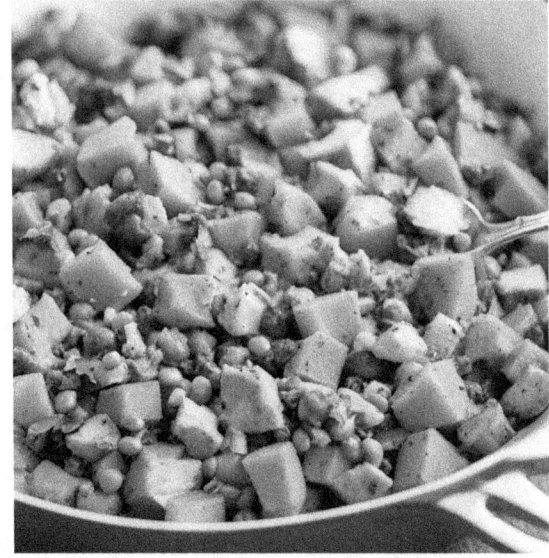

15. Chicken Caprese

Serves: 4
Cooking Time: 25 minutes

Ingredients:
- 4 boneless, skinless chicken breasts
- 2 tablespoons olive oil
- 1 teaspoon dried oregano
- 1 teaspoon garlic powder
- 1 cup cherry tomatoes, halved
- 1/4 cup fresh basil leaves, chopped
- 1/2 cup fresh mozzarella cheese, sliced
- 1 tablespoon balsamic glaze

Instructions:
1. Preheat the oven to 375°F (190°C).
2. In a small bowl, mix together olive oil, dried oregano, and garlic powder. Brush the mixture over the chicken breasts.
3. Heat a large oven-safe skillet over medium-high heat. Add the chicken breasts and cook for about 3-4 minutes on each side, until golden brown.
4. Add the cherry tomatoes to the skillet and transfer to the preheated oven. Bake for 10-12 minutes, until the chicken is cooked through and the internal temperature reaches 165°F (75°C).
5. Remove the skillet from the oven and top each chicken breast with fresh basil and a slice of mozzarella cheese. Return to the oven for an additional 2-3 minutes, until the cheese is melted.
6. Drizzle with balsamic glaze before serving.
7. Serve warm.

Nutrition Information (per serving):
- Calories: 320
- Protein: 35g
- Carbohydrates: 5g
- Dietary Fiber: 1g
- Sugars: 3g
- Fat: 18g
- Saturated Fat: 6g
- Sodium: 200mg

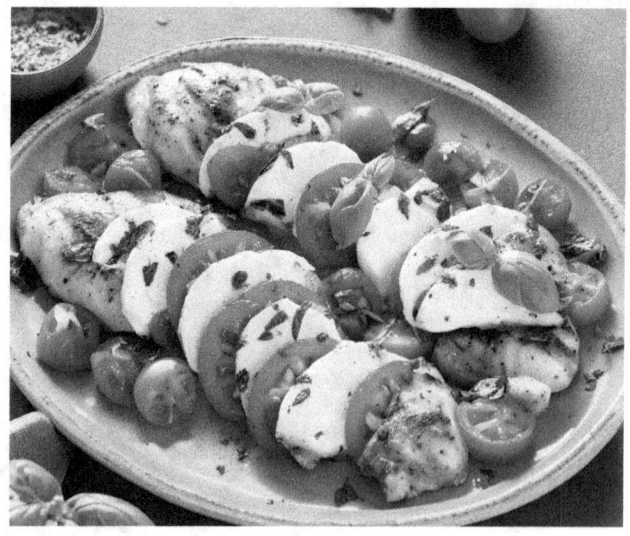

16. Asian Turkey Meatloaf

Serves: 6
Cooking Time: 1 hour
Ingredients:

- 1 pound ground turkey
- 1/2 cup almond flour
- 1 egg, beaten
- 2 cloves garlic, minced
- 1 small onion, finely chopped
- 1/4 cup low-sodium soy sauce
- 1 tablespoon ginger, minced
- 1 tablespoon sesame oil
- 1/4 cup hoisin sauce
- 2 tablespoons rice vinegar
- 1/4 teaspoon crushed red pepper flakes (optional)
- 1/4 cup chopped green onions

Instructions:

1. Preheat the oven to 375°F (190°C). Line a loaf pan with parchment paper.
2. In a large bowl, mix together the ground turkey, almond flour, beaten egg, minced garlic, chopped onion, soy sauce, ginger, sesame oil, and hoisin sauce until well combined.
3. Transfer the mixture to the prepared loaf pan and press down evenly.
4. Bake in the preheated oven for 50-60 minutes, or until the internal temperature reaches 165°F (75°C).
5. In a small bowl, mix together the rice vinegar and crushed red pepper flakes (if using). Brush over the meatloaf during the last 10 minutes of baking.
6. Let the meatloaf rest for 10 minutes before slicing.
7. Garnish with chopped green onions before serving.
8. Serve warm.

Nutrition Information (per serving):

- Calories: 250
- Protein: 20g
- Carbohydrates: 10g
- Dietary Fiber: 2g
- Sugars: 6g
- Fat: 14g
- Saturated Fat: 3g
- Sodium: 350mg

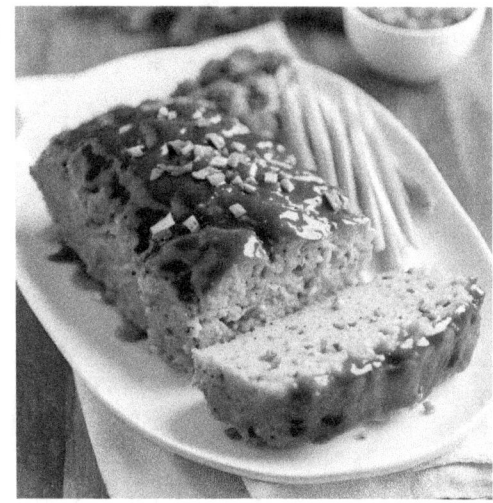

17. Turkey and Spinach Stuffed Shells

Serves: 4
Cooking Time: 40 minutes
Ingredients:

- 12 jumbo pasta shells
- 1 tablespoon olive oil
- 1 pound ground turkey
- 2 cloves garlic, minced
- 2 cups fresh spinach, chopped
- 1 cup ricotta cheese
- 1 egg, beaten
- 1 teaspoon dried basil
- 2 cups marinara sauce
- 1/2 cup shredded mozzarella cheese

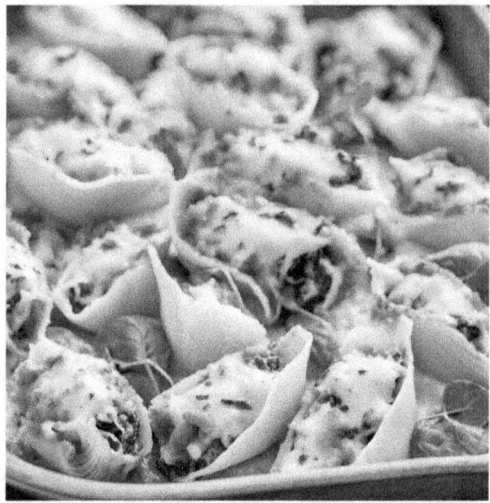

Instructions:

1. Preheat the oven to 375°F (190°C). Lightly grease a baking dish.
2. Cook the pasta shells according to package instructions. Drain and set aside.
3. In a large skillet, heat olive oil over medium heat. Add the ground turkey and cook until browned, about 8-10 minutes.
4. Add the minced garlic and chopped spinach, cooking for another 2-3 minutes, until the spinach is wilted. Remove from heat and let cool slightly.
5. In a large bowl, mix together the ricotta cheese, beaten egg, and dried basil. Stir in the cooked turkey and spinach mixture.
6. Fill each pasta shell with the turkey and spinach mixture and place in the prepared baking dish.
7. Pour the marinara sauce over the stuffed shells and sprinkle with shredded mozzarella cheese.
8. Bake in the preheated oven for 20-25 minutes, until the cheese is melted and bubbly.
9. Serve warm.

Nutrition Information (per serving):

- Calories: 360
- Protein: 30g
- Carbohydrates: 30g
- Dietary Fiber: 5g
- Sugars: 8g
- Fat: 14g
- Saturated Fat: 6g
- Sodium: 480mg

18. Chicken Fajitas

Serves: 4
Cooking Time: 30 minutes
Ingredients:

- 1 pound boneless, skinless chicken breasts, thinly sliced
- 2 tablespoons olive oil
- 1 red bell pepper, sliced
- 1 yellow bell pepper, sliced
- 1 green bell pepper, sliced
- 1 large onion, sliced
- 1 teaspoon garlic powder
- 1 teaspoon ground cumin
- 1 teaspoon chili powder
- 1 tablespoon lime juice
- 8 small whole wheat tortillas
- 1/4 cup chopped fresh cilantro

Instructions:

1. In a large skillet, heat 1 tablespoon of olive oil over medium-high heat. Add the sliced chicken breasts and cook until no longer pink, about 5-7 minutes. Remove from skillet and set aside.
2. Add the remaining 1 tablespoon of olive oil to the skillet. Add the red, yellow, and green bell peppers, and onion. Cook for about 7-10 minutes, until the vegetables are tender.
3. Return the cooked chicken to the skillet and stir in the garlic powder, ground cumin, chili powder, and lime juice. Cook for an additional 2-3 minutes, until everything is heated through.
4. Warm the whole wheat tortillas in a dry skillet or microwave.
5. Serve the chicken and vegetable mixture in the tortillas, garnished with chopped fresh cilantro.
6. Serve warm.

Nutrition Information (per serving):

- Calories: 350
- Protein: 28g
- Carbohydrates: 30g
- Dietary Fiber: 6g
- Sugars: 6g
- Fat: 12g
- Saturated Fat: 2.5g
- Sodium: 300mg

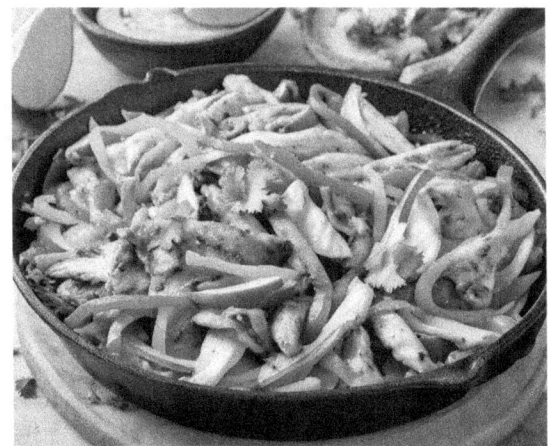

19. Turkey and Cabbage Stir-fry

Serves: 4
Cooking Time: 20 minutes
Ingredients:
- 2 tablespoons olive oil
- 1 pound ground turkey
- 1 small onion, diced
- 2 cloves garlic, minced
- 1 small head of cabbage, shredded
- 1 carrot, grated
- 3 tablespoons low-sodium soy sauce
- 1 tablespoon rice vinegar
- 1 tablespoon honey or maple syrup (optional)
- 1/4 teaspoon crushed red pepper flakes (optional)

Instructions:
1. Heat olive oil in a large skillet over medium heat. Add the ground turkey and cook until browned, about 8-10 minutes.
2. Add the diced onion and minced garlic, cooking until softened, about 5 minutes.
3. Stir in the shredded cabbage and grated carrot, cooking for another 5-7 minutes, until the vegetables are tender.
4. In a small bowl, mix together the soy sauce, rice vinegar, honey or maple syrup (if using), and crushed red pepper flakes (if using).
5. Pour the sauce over the turkey and vegetable mixture, stirring to combine. Cook for an additional 2-3 minutes, until everything is heated through.
6. Serve warm.

Nutrition Information (per serving):
- Calories: 250
- Protein: 24g
- Carbohydrates: 14g
- Dietary Fiber: 4g
- Sugars: 6g
- Fat: 12g
- Saturated Fat: 2.5g
- Sodium: 350mg

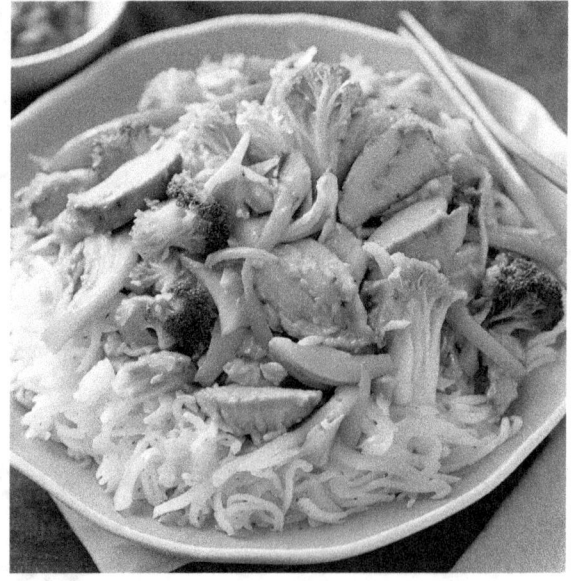

20. Balsamic Glazed Chicken Breast

Serves: 4
Cooking Time: 25 minutes
Ingredients:
- 4 boneless, skinless chicken breasts
- 2 tablespoons olive oil
- 1/4 cup balsamic vinegar
- 2 cloves garlic, minced
- 1 tablespoon honey or maple syrup
- 1 teaspoon dried thyme

Instructions:
1. Preheat the oven to 375°F (190°C).
2. In a small bowl, mix together the balsamic vinegar, minced garlic, honey or maple syrup, and dried thyme.
3. Heat olive oil in an oven-safe skillet over medium-high heat. Add the chicken breasts and cook for about 3-4 minutes on each side, until golden brown.
4. Pour the balsamic glaze over the chicken breasts.
5. Transfer the skillet to the preheated oven and bake for 15-20 minutes, or until the chicken is cooked through and the internal temperature reaches 165°F (75°C).
6. Let the chicken rest for 5 minutes before serving.
7. Serve warm.

Nutrition Information (per serving):
- Calories: 280
- Protein: 35g
- Carbohydrates: 10g
- Dietary Fiber: 0g
- Sugars: 7g
- Fat: 10g
- Saturated Fat: 2g
- Sodium: 180mg

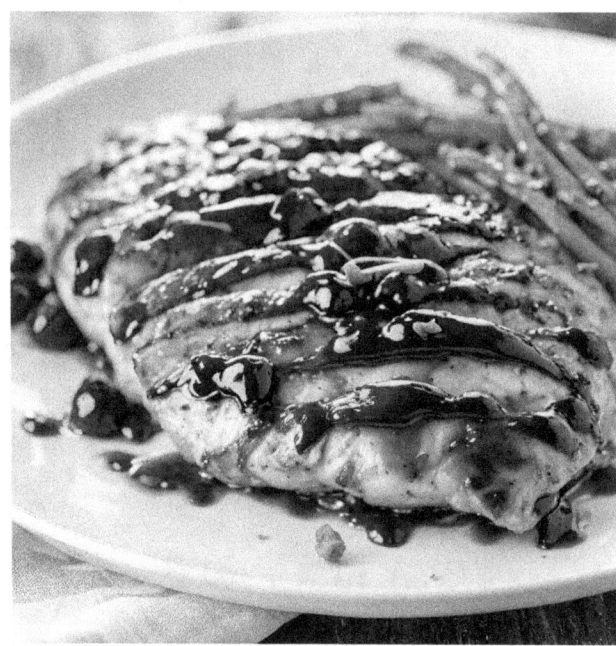

21. Pesto Turkey Pinwheels

Serves: 4
Cooking Time: 20 minutes
Ingredients:
- 4 whole wheat tortillas
- 1/2 cup basil pesto
- 1 pound sliced turkey breast
- 1 cup baby spinach
- 1/2 cup roasted red peppers, sliced

Instructions:
1. Lay the whole wheat tortillas flat on a clean surface.
2. Spread 2 tablespoons of basil pesto evenly over each tortilla.
3. Layer the sliced turkey breast, baby spinach, and roasted red peppers over the pesto.
4. Roll each tortilla tightly and slice into pinwheels.
5. Serve immediately or refrigerate for up to 1 day.

Nutrition Information (per serving):
- Calories: 300
- Protein: 25g
- Carbohydrates: 25g
- Dietary Fiber: 5g
- Sugars: 3g
- Fat: 12g
- Saturated Fat: 2g
- Sodium: 480mg

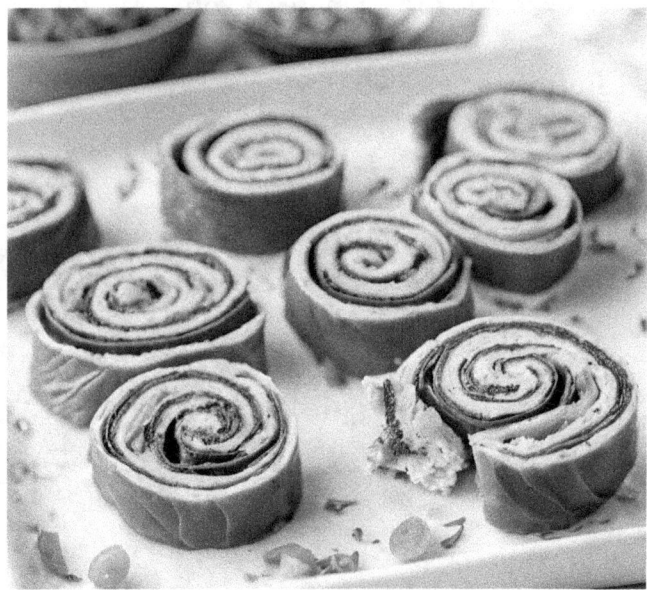

22. Roasted Chicken with Root Vegetables

Serves: 4
Cooking Time: 1 hour 15 minutes
Ingredients:
- 4 bone-in, skin-on chicken thighs
- 2 tablespoons olive oil
- 1 teaspoon dried rosemary
- 1 teaspoon dried thyme
- 1 tablespoon lemon juice
- 1 pound carrots, peeled and cut into chunks
- 1 pound parsnips, peeled and cut into chunks
- 1 large sweet potato, peeled and cut into chunks
- 1 small red onion, cut into wedges

Instructions:
1. Preheat the oven to 400°F (200°C). Line a baking sheet with parchment paper.
2. In a small bowl, mix together 1 tablespoon of olive oil, dried rosemary, dried thyme, and lemon juice. Rub the mixture over the chicken thighs.
3. In a large bowl, toss the carrots, parsnips, sweet potato, and red onion with the remaining 1 tablespoon of olive oil.
4. Spread the vegetables in a single layer on the prepared baking sheet. Place the chicken thighs on top of the vegetables.
5. Roast in the preheated oven for 60-75 minutes, or until the chicken is cooked through and the vegetables are tender.
6. Let the chicken rest for 5 minutes before serving.
7. Serve warm.

Nutrition Information (per serving):
- Calories: 380
- Protein: 25g
- Carbohydrates: 35g
- Dietary Fiber: 8g
- Sugars: 10g
- Fat: 18g
- Saturated Fat: 4g
- Sodium: 200mg

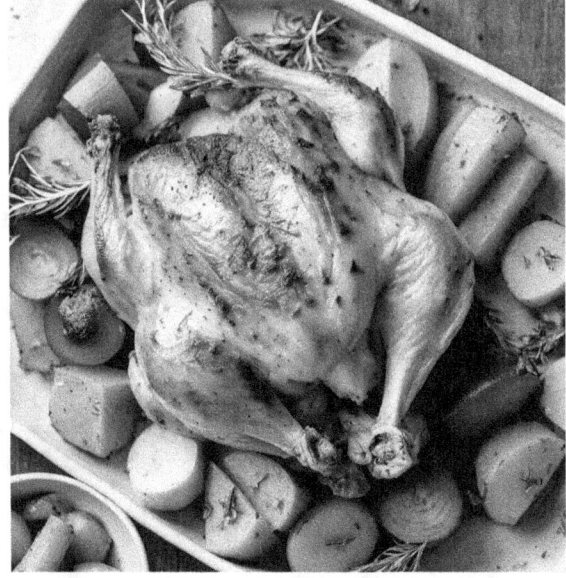

23. Smoked Paprika Turkey Legs

Serves: 4
Cooking Time: 1 hour 15 minutes
Ingredients:
- 4 turkey legs
- 2 tablespoons olive oil
- 2 teaspoons smoked paprika
- 1 teaspoon garlic powder
- 1 teaspoon onion powder
- 1 tablespoon lemon juice

Instructions:
1. Preheat the oven to 375°F (190°C).
2. In a small bowl, mix together the olive oil, smoked paprika, garlic powder, onion powder, and lemon juice.
3. Rub the mixture all over the turkey legs.
4. Place the turkey legs in a roasting pan.
5. Roast in the preheated oven for 75 minutes, or until the internal temperature reaches 165°F (75°C).
6. Let the turkey legs rest for 10 minutes before serving.
7. Serve warm.

Nutrition Information (per serving):
- Calories: 350
- Protein: 40g
- Carbohydrates: 1g
- Dietary Fiber: 0g
- Sugars: 0g
- Fat: 20g
- Saturated Fat: 4g
- Sodium: 80mg

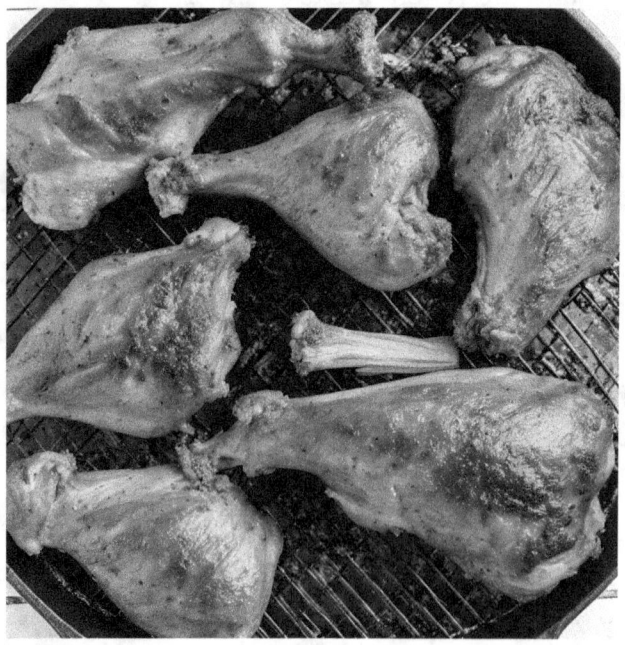

24. Chicken Bruschetta

Serves: 4
Cooking Time: 30 minutes
Ingredients:
- 4 boneless, skinless chicken breasts
- 2 tablespoons olive oil, divided
- 1 teaspoon dried oregano
- 1 teaspoon garlic powder
- 2 cups cherry tomatoes, halved
- 1/4 cup red onion, finely chopped
- 2 cloves garlic, minced
- 1/4 cup fresh basil leaves, chopped
- 1 tablespoon balsamic vinegar

Instructions:
1. Preheat the oven to 375°F (190°C).
2. In a small bowl, mix together 1 tablespoon of olive oil, dried oregano, and garlic powder. Brush the mixture over the chicken breasts.
3. Heat the remaining 1 tablespoon of olive oil in an oven-safe skillet over medium-high heat. Add the chicken breasts and cook for about 3-4 minutes on each side, until golden brown.
4. Transfer the skillet to the preheated oven and bake for 15-20 minutes, or until the chicken is cooked through and the internal temperature reaches 165°F (75°C).
5. While the chicken is baking, combine the cherry tomatoes, red onion, minced garlic, fresh basil, and balsamic vinegar in a bowl. Toss to mix well.
6. Once the chicken is done, top each breast with the tomato mixture.
7. Serve warm.

Nutrition Information (per serving):
- Calories: 280
- Protein: 35g
- Carbohydrates: 10g
- Dietary Fiber: 2g
- Sugars: 5g
- Fat: 12g
- Saturated Fat: 2g
- Sodium: 180mg

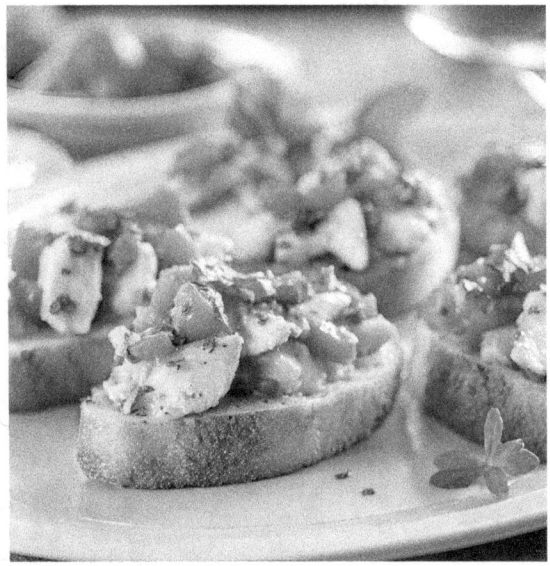

25. Chicken and Asparagus Stir-fry

Serves: 4
Cooking Time: 20 minutes

Ingredients:
- 2 tablespoons olive oil
- 1 pound boneless, skinless chicken breasts, thinly sliced
- 2 cloves garlic, minced
- 1 tablespoon fresh ginger, minced
- 1 bunch asparagus, cut into 2-inch pieces
- 1 red bell pepper, sliced
- 3 tablespoons low-sodium soy sauce
- 1 tablespoon rice vinegar
- 1 tablespoon honey or maple syrup (optional)
- 1/4 teaspoon crushed red pepper flakes (optional)

Instructions:
1. Heat 1 tablespoon of olive oil in a large skillet or wok over medium-high heat. Add the sliced chicken and cook until no longer pink, about 5-7 minutes. Remove from skillet and set aside.
2. Add the remaining 1 tablespoon of olive oil to the skillet. Add the minced garlic and ginger, cooking for 1-2 minutes until fragrant.
3. Add the asparagus and red bell pepper, stir-frying for about 5-7 minutes, until the vegetables are tender-crisp.
4. Return the cooked chicken to the skillet.
5. In a small bowl, mix together the soy sauce, rice vinegar, honey or maple syrup (if using), and crushed red pepper flakes (if using). Pour the sauce over the chicken and vegetables, stirring to combine.
6. Cook for another 2-3 minutes, until everything is heated through.
7. Serve warm.

Nutrition Information (per serving):
- Calories: 280
- Protein: 30g
- Carbohydrates: 12g
- Dietary Fiber: 3g
- Sugars: 5g
- Fat: 12g
- Saturated Fat: 2g
- Sodium: 320mg

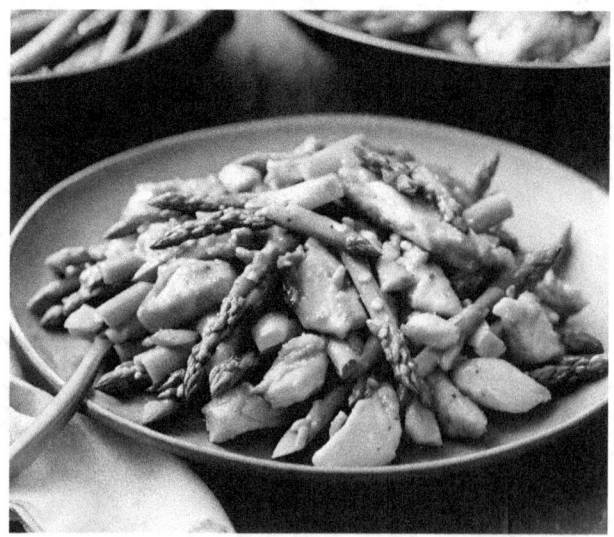

26. Lemon and Thyme Turkey Cutlets

Serves: 4
Cooking Time: 20 minutes
Ingredients:

- 4 turkey cutlets
- 2 tablespoons olive oil
- 2 cloves garlic, minced
- 1 teaspoon dried thyme
- 1 tablespoon lemon zest
- 1 tablespoon lemon juice

Instructions:

1. In a small bowl, mix together the olive oil, minced garlic, dried thyme, lemon zest, and lemon juice.
2. Rub the mixture all over the turkey cutlets.
3. Heat a large skillet over medium-high heat. Add the turkey cutlets and cook for about 4-5 minutes on each side, until golden brown and cooked through.
4. Remove from heat and let rest for a few minutes before serving.
5. Serve warm.

Nutrition Information (per serving):

- Calories: 240
- Protein: 30g
- Carbohydrates: 2g
- Dietary Fiber: 0g
- Sugars: 0g
- Fat: 12g
- Saturated Fat: 2.5g
- Sodium: 90mg

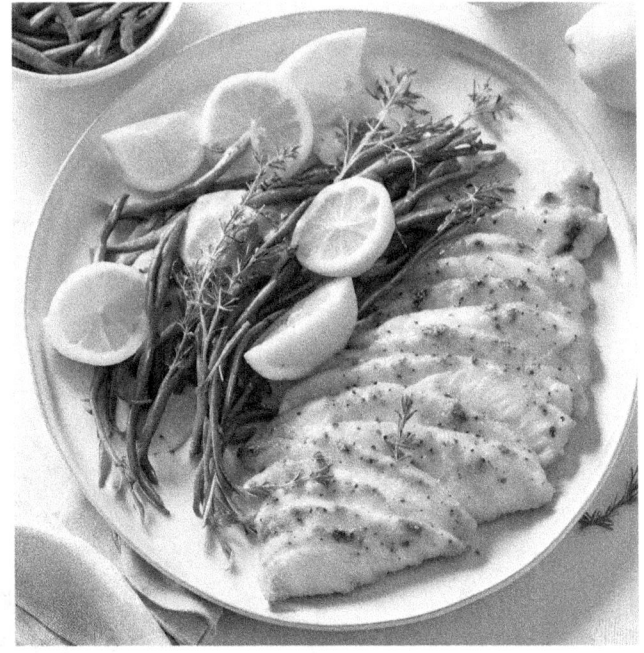

Fish Recipes

1. Grilled Salmon with Lemon and Herbs
Serves: 4
Cooking Time: 20 minutes
Ingredients:
- 4 salmon fillets (about 6 oz each)
- 3 tablespoons olive oil
- 2 tablespoons lemon juice
- 2 cloves garlic, minced
- 1 teaspoon dried thyme
- 1 teaspoon dried rosemary
- 1 tablespoon lemon zest
- Lemon slices for garnish
- Fresh parsley for garnish

Instructions:
1. Preheat the grill to medium-high heat.
2. In a small bowl, mix together the olive oil, lemon juice, minced garlic, dried thyme, dried rosemary, and lemon zest.
3. Brush the mixture over the salmon fillets.
4. Grill the salmon fillets for about 5-6 minutes on each side, or until the fish is cooked through and flakes easily with a fork.
5. Garnish with lemon slices and fresh parsley before serving.
6. Serve warm.

Nutrition Information (per serving):
- Calories: 350
- Protein: 34g
- Carbohydrates: 2g
- Dietary Fiber: 0g
- Sugars: 0g
- Fat: 22g
- Saturated Fat: 4g
- Sodium: 75mg

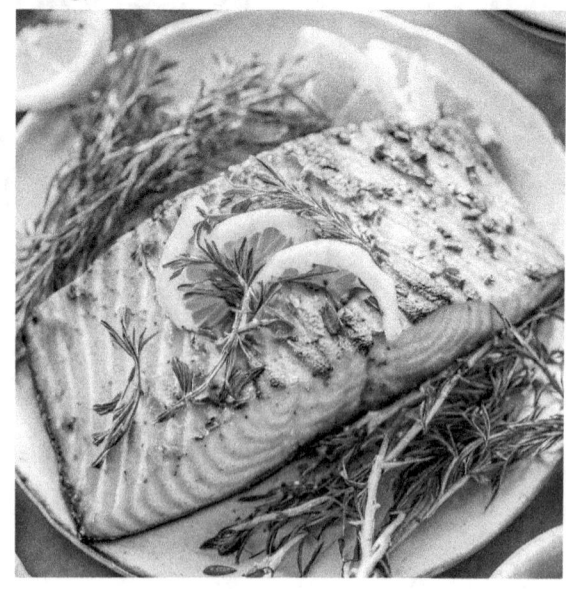

2. **Baked Cod with Olive Tapenade**
Serves: 4
Cooking Time: 25 minutes
Ingredients:
- 4 cod fillets (about 6 oz each)
- 2 tablespoons olive oil
- 1 cup pitted Kalamata olives
- 2 cloves garlic, minced
- 1 tablespoon capers
- 1 tablespoon lemon juice
- 1 teaspoon dried oregano
- 1/4 cup chopped fresh parsley

Instructions:
1. Preheat the oven to 400°F (200°C). Line a baking dish with parchment paper.
2. In a food processor, combine the olives, garlic, capers, lemon juice, dried oregano, and 1 tablespoon of olive oil. Pulse until finely chopped and well combined.
3. Place the cod fillets in the prepared baking dish. Drizzle with the remaining 1 tablespoon of olive oil.
4. Spread the olive tapenade evenly over the top of each cod fillet.
5. Bake in the preheated oven for 15-20 minutes, or until the fish is opaque and flakes easily with a fork.
6. Garnish with chopped fresh parsley before serving.
7. Serve warm.

Nutrition Information (per serving):
- Calories: 280
- Protein: 28g
- Carbohydrates: 3g
- Dietary Fiber: 1g
- Sugars: 0g
- Fat: 18g
- Saturated Fat: 3g
- Sodium: 400mg

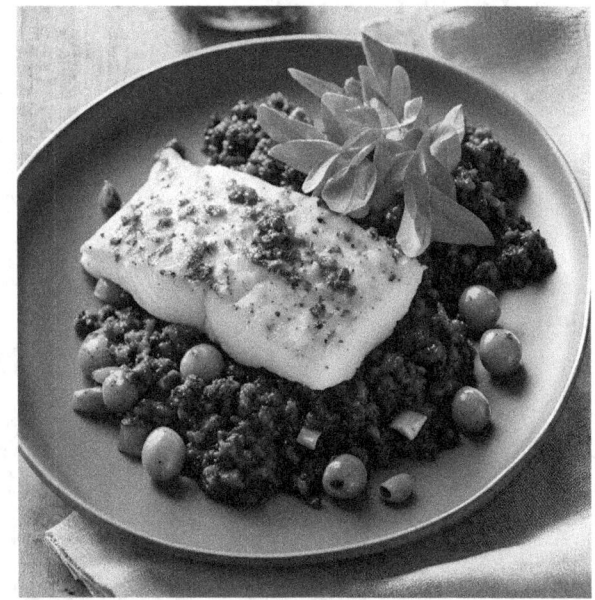

3. Asian-Inspired Tuna Poke Bowl

Serves: 4
Cooking Time: 20 minutes
Ingredients:
- 1 pound sushi-grade tuna, diced
- 1/4 cup low-sodium soy sauce
- 1 tablespoon sesame oil
- 1 tablespoon rice vinegar
- 1 tablespoon honey or maple syrup (optional)
- 1 teaspoon fresh ginger, minced
- 2 cups cooked brown rice
- 1 avocado, diced
- 1 cucumber, sliced
- 1 carrot, grated
- 1/4 cup sliced green onions
- 1 tablespoon sesame seeds

Instructions:
1. In a medium bowl, combine the soy sauce, sesame oil, rice vinegar, honey or maple syrup (if using), and minced ginger.
2. Add the diced tuna to the bowl and toss to coat. Let marinate for at least 10 minutes.
3. Divide the cooked brown rice among four bowls.
4. Top each bowl with marinated tuna, avocado, cucumber, carrot, and sliced green onions.
5. Sprinkle with sesame seeds before serving.
6. Serve immediately.

Nutrition Information (per serving):
- Calories: 420
- Protein: 28g
- Carbohydrates: 45g
- Dietary Fiber: 8g
- Sugars: 7g
- Fat: 16g
- Saturated Fat: 2.5g
- Sodium: 480mg

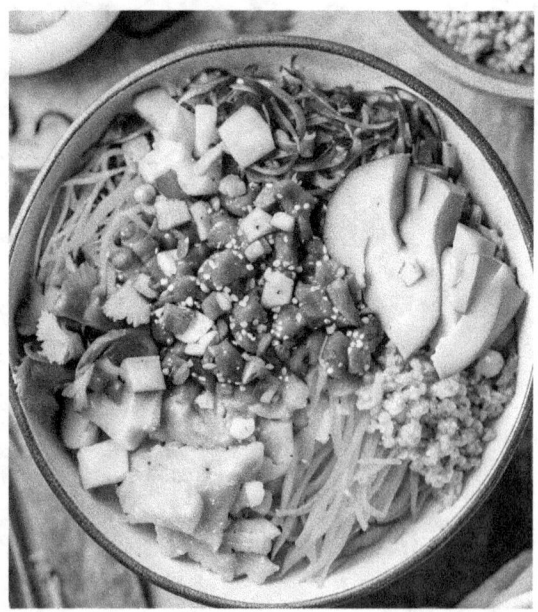

4. Sardines in Tomato Sauce

Serves: 4
Cooking Time: 30 minutes
Ingredients:

- 2 tablespoons olive oil
- 1 small onion, finely chopped
- 2 cloves garlic, minced
- 1 can (14 oz) diced tomatoes
- 1 tablespoon tomato paste
- 1 teaspoon dried basil
- 1 teaspoon dried oregano
- 1 tablespoon lemon juice
- 4 cans (3.75 oz each) sardines in water, drained
- Fresh parsley for garnish

Instructions:

1. In a large skillet, heat olive oil over medium heat. Add the finely chopped onion and minced garlic, cooking until softened, about 5 minutes.
2. Stir in the diced tomatoes, tomato paste, dried basil, dried oregano, and lemon juice. Bring to a simmer and cook for 15-20 minutes, until the sauce thickens.
3. Add the sardines to the skillet, gently stirring to coat with the tomato sauce. Cook for an additional 5 minutes, until the sardines are heated through.
4. Garnish with fresh parsley before serving.
5. Serve warm.

Nutrition Information (per serving):

- Calories: 240
- Protein: 20g
- Carbohydrates: 10g
- Dietary Fiber: 2g
- Sugars: 5g
- Fat: 14g
- Saturated Fat: 2g
- Sodium: 400mg

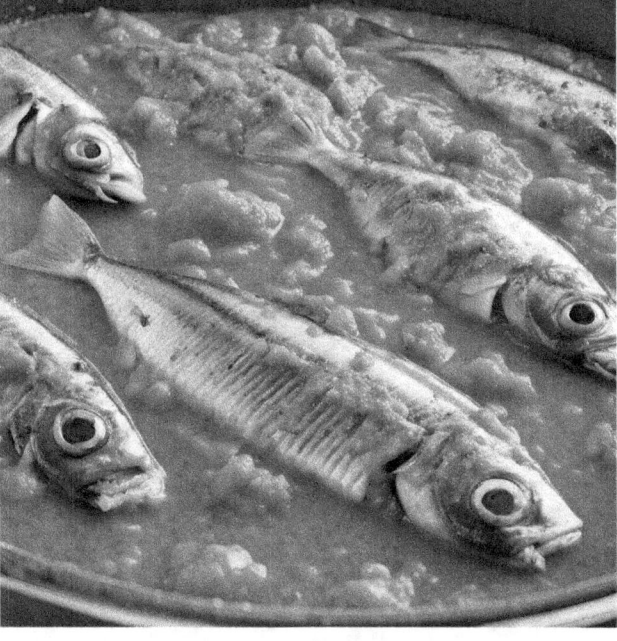

5. Herb-Crusted Tilapia

Serves: 4
Cooking Time: 20 minutes
Ingredients:
- 4 tilapia fillets (about 6 oz each)
- 1/2 cup almond flour
- 1 tablespoon dried parsley
- 1 teaspoon dried thyme
- 1 teaspoon garlic powder
- 2 tablespoons olive oil
- 1 tablespoon lemon juice

Instructions:
1. Preheat the oven to 400°F (200°C). Line a baking sheet with parchment paper.
2. In a shallow dish, mix the almond flour, dried parsley, dried thyme, and garlic powder.
3. Brush the tilapia fillets with olive oil, then dredge them in the herb mixture, pressing gently to coat.
4. Place the coated tilapia fillets on the prepared baking sheet.
5. Bake in the preheated oven for 15-20 minutes, or until the fish is opaque and flakes easily with a fork.
6. Drizzle with lemon juice before serving.
7. Serve warm.

Nutrition Information (per serving):
- Calories: 280
- Protein: 30g
- Carbohydrates: 4g
- Dietary Fiber: 2g
- Sugars: 1g
- Fat: 16g
- Saturated Fat: 2.5g
- Sodium: 80mg

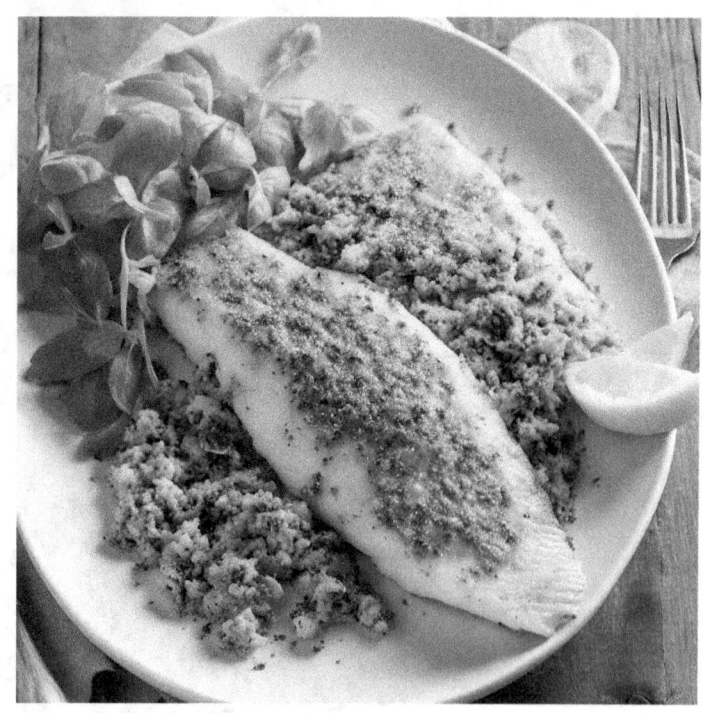

6. Mackerel Salad

Serves: 4
Cooking Time: 15 minutes
Ingredients:
- 2 cans (5 oz each) mackerel in water, drained and flaked
- 1 cup cherry tomatoes, halved
- 1 cucumber, diced
- 1/4 cup red onion, finely chopped
- 1/4 cup fresh parsley, chopped
- 3 tablespoons olive oil
- 2 tablespoons lemon juice
- 1 teaspoon dried oregano

Instructions:
1. In a large bowl, combine the flaked mackerel, cherry tomatoes, cucumber, red onion, and fresh parsley.
2. In a small bowl, whisk together the olive oil, lemon juice, and dried oregano.
3. Pour the dressing over the mackerel mixture and toss to combine.
4. Serve immediately or refrigerate for up to 1 day.

Nutrition Information (per serving):
- Calories: 250
- Protein: 20g
- Carbohydrates: 6g
- Dietary Fiber: 2g
- Sugars: 3g
- Fat: 18g
- Saturated Fat: 3g
- Sodium: 300mg

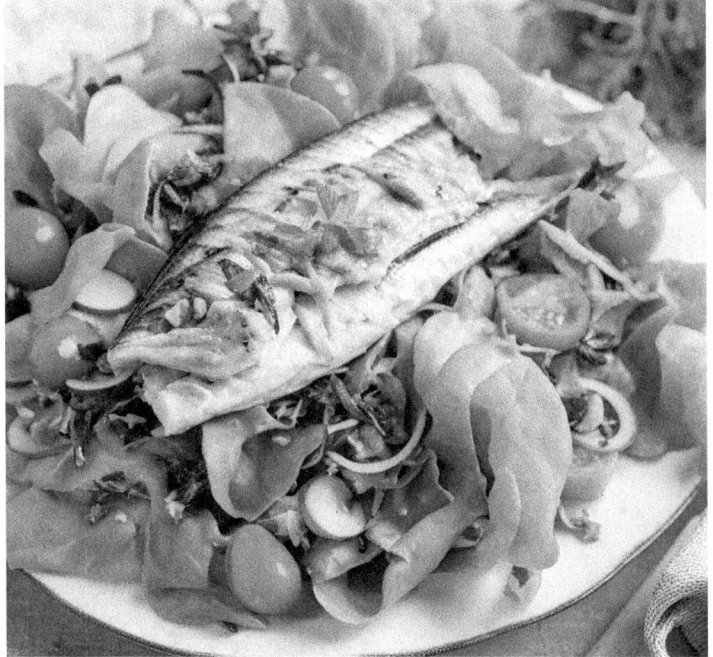

7. Trout Almondine

Serves: 4
Cooking Time: 20 minutes
Ingredients:
- 4 trout fillets (about 6 oz each)
- 1/4 cup almond flour
- 2 tablespoons olive oil
- 1/4 cup sliced almonds
- 2 tablespoons lemon juice
- 1 tablespoon fresh parsley, chopped

Instructions:
1. Preheat the oven to 375°F (190°C). Line a baking sheet with parchment paper.
2. Dredge the trout fillets in almond flour, shaking off any excess.
3. In a large skillet, heat olive oil over medium heat. Add the trout fillets and cook for 3-4 minutes on each side, until golden brown and cooked through.
4. Transfer the cooked trout fillets to the prepared baking sheet and keep warm in the oven.
5. In the same skillet, add the sliced almonds and cook until golden, about 2 minutes.
6. Stir in the lemon juice and chopped parsley, and cook for an additional minute.
7. Pour the almond mixture over the trout fillets.
8. Serve warm.

Nutrition Information (per serving):
- Calories: 350
- Protein: 32g
- Carbohydrates: 4g
- Dietary Fiber: 2g
- Sugars: 1g
- Fat: 22g
- Saturated Fat: 3.5g
- Sodium: 90mg

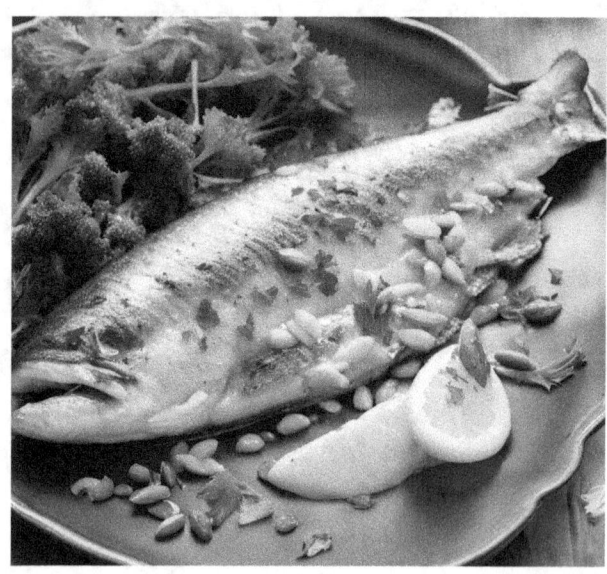

8. Spicy Grilled Shrimp

Serves: 4
Cooking Time: 15 minutes
Ingredients:
- 1 pound large shrimp, peeled and deveined
- 2 tablespoons olive oil
- 1 tablespoon lemon juice
- 2 cloves garlic, minced
- 1 teaspoon paprika
- 1/2 teaspoon cayenne pepper
- 1/2 teaspoon garlic powder
- 1 tablespoon fresh cilantro, chopped

Instructions:
1. Preheat the grill to medium-high heat.
2. In a large bowl, combine the olive oil, lemon juice, minced garlic, paprika, cayenne pepper, and garlic powder.
3. Add the shrimp to the bowl and toss to coat evenly.
4. Thread the shrimp onto skewers.
5. Grill the shrimp for about 2-3 minutes on each side, until opaque and cooked through.
6. Remove from the grill and sprinkle with chopped fresh cilantro.
7. Serve immediately.

Nutrition Information (per serving):
- Calories: 180
- Protein: 24g
- Carbohydrates: 2g
- Dietary Fiber: 1g
- Sugars: 0g
- Fat: 8g
- Saturated Fat: 1.5g
- Sodium: 320mg

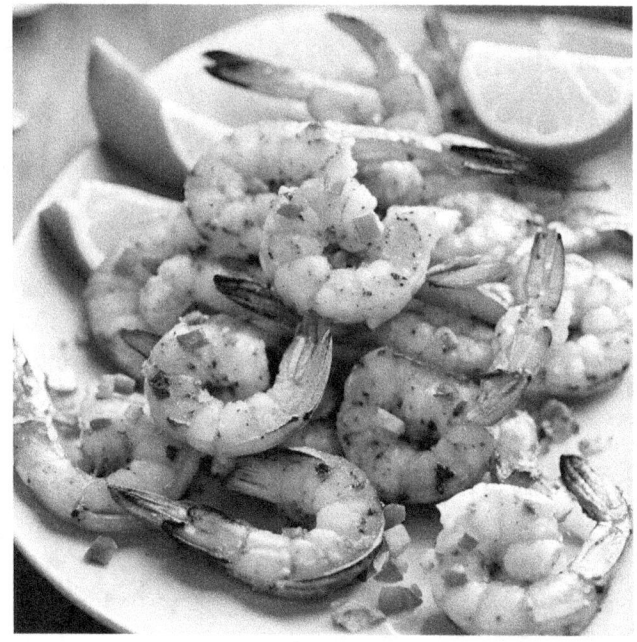

9. Lemon Butter Haddock

Serves: 4
Cooking Time: 20 minutes

Ingredients:
- 4 haddock fillets (about 6 oz each)
- 2 tablespoons olive oil
- 2 tablespoons unsalted butter
- 2 cloves garlic, minced
- 1 tablespoon lemon zest
- 2 tablespoons lemon juice
- 1 tablespoon fresh parsley, chopped

Instructions:
1. Preheat the oven to 375°F (190°C). Line a baking dish with parchment paper.
2. In a small saucepan, melt the butter over medium heat. Add the minced garlic and cook for 1-2 minutes until fragrant. Stir in the lemon zest and lemon juice.
3. Place the haddock fillets in the prepared baking dish. Drizzle with olive oil and the lemon butter sauce.
4. Bake in the preheated oven for 15-20 minutes, or until the fish is opaque and flakes easily with a fork.
5. Garnish with chopped fresh parsley before serving.
6. Serve warm.

Nutrition Information (per serving):
- Calories: 260
- Protein: 30g
- Carbohydrates: 2g
- Dietary Fiber: 0g
- Sugars: 0g
- Fat: 14g
- Saturated Fat: 5g
- Sodium: 90mg

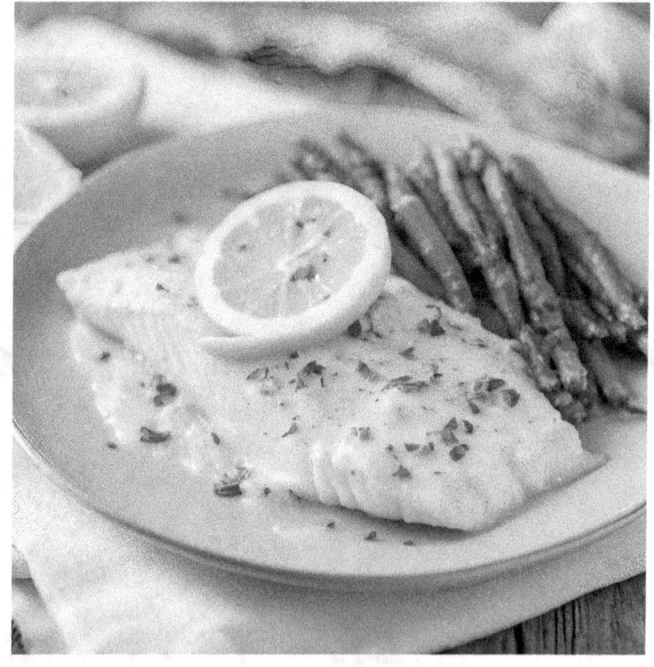

10. Salmon and Quinoa Salad

Serves: 4
Cooking Time: 25 minutes
Ingredients:

- 4 salmon fillets (about 6 oz each)
- 1 cup quinoa, rinsed
- 2 cups water
- 1 cup cherry tomatoes, halved
- 1 cucumber, diced
- 1/4 cup red onion, finely chopped
- 1/4 cup fresh parsley, chopped
- 3 tablespoons olive oil
- 2 tablespoons lemon juice
- 1 teaspoon dried oregano

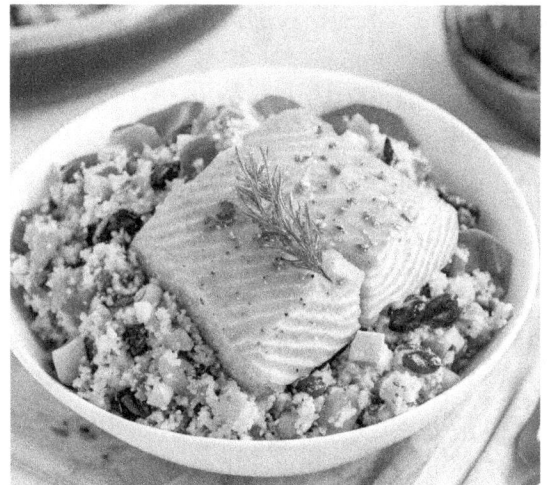

Instructions:

1. Preheat the oven to 375°F (190°C). Line a baking sheet with parchment paper.
2. Place the salmon fillets on the prepared baking sheet. Drizzle with 1 tablespoon of olive oil and 1 tablespoon of lemon juice.
3. Bake in the preheated oven for 15-20 minutes, or until the salmon is cooked through and flakes easily with a fork.
4. While the salmon is baking, bring the water to a boil in a medium saucepan. Add the quinoa, reduce heat to low, and simmer for 15 minutes or until the water is absorbed. Fluff with a fork and let cool slightly.
5. In a large bowl, combine the cooked quinoa, cherry tomatoes, cucumber, red onion, and fresh parsley.
6. In a small bowl, whisk together the remaining 2 tablespoons of olive oil, 1 tablespoon of lemon juice, and dried oregano. Pour over the quinoa mixture and toss to combine.
7. Top the quinoa salad with the baked salmon fillets.
8. Serve warm or chilled.

Nutrition Information (per serving):

- Calories: 450
- Protein: 35g
- Carbohydrates: 30g
- Dietary Fiber: 5g
- Sugars: 3g
- Fat: 22g
- Saturated Fat: 4g
- Sodium: 120mg

11. Halibut Steaks with Mango Salsa

Serves: 4
Cooking Time: 20 minutes

Ingredients:
- 4 halibut steaks (about 6 oz each)
- 2 tablespoons olive oil
- 1 tablespoon lemon juice
- 1 mango, diced
- 1/2 red bell pepper, diced
- 1/4 cup red onion, finely chopped
- 1 tablespoon fresh cilantro, chopped
- 1 tablespoon lime juice

Instructions:
1. Preheat the grill to medium-high heat.
2. Brush the halibut steaks with olive oil and drizzle with lemon juice.
3. Grill the halibut steaks for about 5-6 minutes on each side, or until the fish is opaque and flakes easily with a fork.
4. While the halibut is grilling, combine the diced mango, red bell pepper, red onion, fresh cilantro, and lime juice in a bowl. Toss to combine.
5. Serve the grilled halibut steaks topped with mango salsa.
6. Serve warm.

Nutrition Information (per serving):
- Calories: 350
- Protein: 35g
- Carbohydrates: 12g
- Dietary Fiber: 2g
- Sugars: 8g
- Fat: 18g
- Saturated Fat: 3g
- Sodium: 100mg

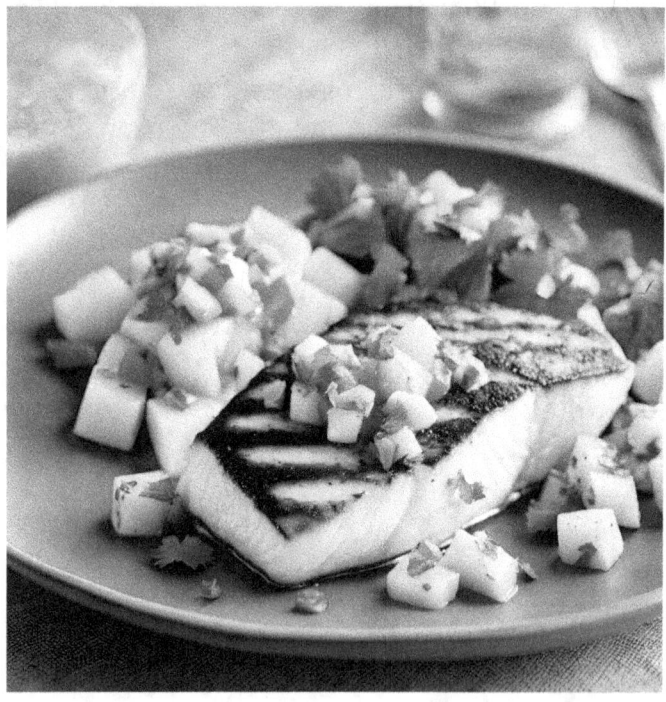

12. Sea Bass with Fennel and Orange

Serves: 4
Cooking Time: 30 minutes
Ingredients:

- 4 sea bass fillets (about 6 oz each)
- 2 tablespoons olive oil
- 1 bulb fennel, thinly sliced
- 1 orange, thinly sliced
- 2 cloves garlic, minced
- 1 tablespoon fresh thyme leaves
- 1 tablespoon orange zest

Instructions:

1. Preheat the oven to 375°F (190°C). Line a baking dish with parchment paper.
2. In a large bowl, toss the sliced fennel, orange slices, minced garlic, and fresh thyme with 1 tablespoon of olive oil.
3. Place the sea bass fillets in the prepared baking dish. Arrange the fennel and orange mixture around the fish.
4. Drizzle the remaining 1 tablespoon of olive oil over the fish and sprinkle with orange zest.
5. Bake in the preheated oven for 20-25 minutes, or until the fish is opaque and flakes easily with a fork.
6. Serve warm.

Nutrition Information (per serving):

- Calories: 320
- Protein: 32g
- Carbohydrates: 8g
- Dietary Fiber: 2g
- Sugars: 4g
- Fat: 18g
- Saturated Fat: 3g
- Sodium: 90mg

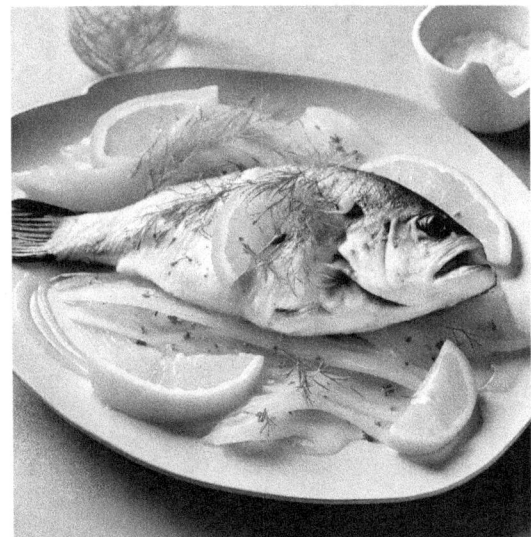

13. Smoked Salmon Frittata

Serves: 4
Cooking Time: 30 minutes
Ingredients:
- 8 large eggs
- 1/4 cup unsweetened almond milk
- 1 tablespoon olive oil
- 1 small red onion, thinly sliced
- 1 cup baby spinach
- 4 oz smoked salmon, chopped
- 1/4 cup fresh dill, chopped
- 1 tablespoon capers, rinsed

Instructions:
1. Preheat the oven to 350°F (175°C).
2. In a large bowl, whisk together the eggs and almond milk.
3. Heat the olive oil in an oven-safe skillet over medium heat. Add the sliced red onion and cook until softened, about 5 minutes.
4. Add the baby spinach to the skillet and cook until wilted, about 2 minutes.
5. Pour the egg mixture into the skillet and stir to combine with the vegetables.
6. Add the chopped smoked salmon, fresh dill, and capers, distributing evenly throughout the egg mixture.
7. Cook on the stovetop for about 5 minutes, until the edges start to set.
8. Transfer the skillet to the preheated oven and bake for 15-20 minutes, or until the frittata is fully set and golden on top.
9. Let the frittata cool slightly before slicing.
10. Serve warm.

Nutrition Information (per serving):
- Calories: 220
- Protein: 20g
- Carbohydrates: 4g
- Dietary Fiber: 1g
- Sugars: 1g
- Fat: 14g
- Saturated Fat: 3g
- Sodium: 480mg

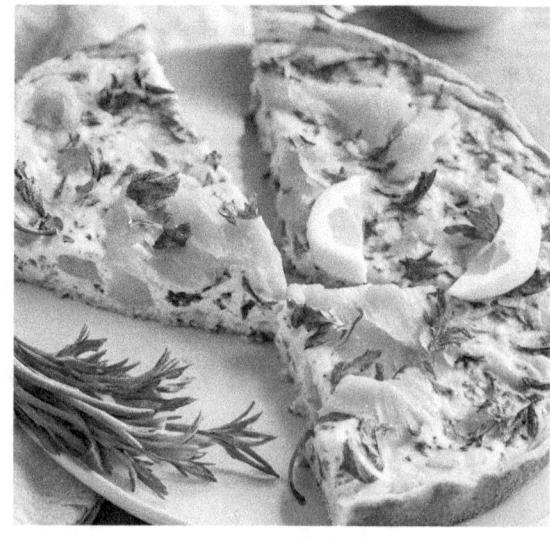

14. Panko-Crusted Sole

Serves: 4
Cooking Time: 20 minutes
Ingredients:
- 4 sole fillets (about 6 oz each)
- 1 cup panko breadcrumbs
- 2 tablespoons olive oil
- 1 teaspoon garlic powder
- 1 teaspoon dried parsley
- 1 tablespoon lemon zest
- 2 tablespoons Dijon mustard
- Lemon wedges for serving

Instructions:
1. Preheat the oven to 400°F (200°C). Line a baking sheet with parchment paper.
2. In a shallow dish, combine panko breadcrumbs, garlic powder, dried parsley, and lemon zest.
3. Brush the sole fillets with Dijon mustard.
4. Press each fillet into the breadcrumb mixture, coating both sides evenly.
5. Place the coated fillets on the prepared baking sheet. Drizzle with olive oil.
6. Bake in the preheated oven for 12-15 minutes, or until the fish is golden brown and flakes easily with a fork.
7. Serve with lemon wedges.

Nutrition Information (per serving):
- Calories: 320
- Protein: 28g
- Carbohydrates: 16g
- Dietary Fiber: 2g
- Sugars: 1g
- Fat: 16g
- Saturated Fat: 2.5g
- Sodium: 220mg

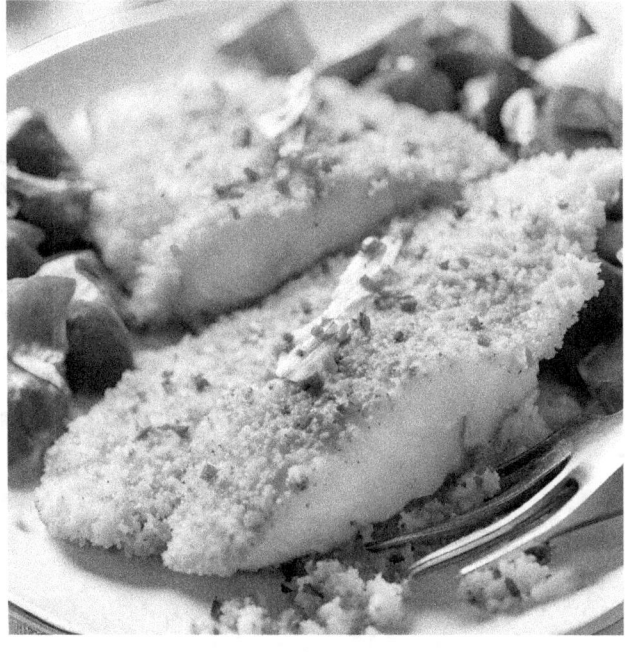

15. Scallops with Pea Puree

Serves: 4

Cooking Time: 20 minutes

Ingredients:
- 1 pound sea scallops
- 2 tablespoons olive oil
- 2 cups frozen peas, thawed
- 1/2 cup unsweetened almond milk
- 2 cloves garlic, minced
- 1 tablespoon lemon juice
- 1 tablespoon fresh mint, chopped

Instructions:
1. In a blender or food processor, combine the thawed peas, almond milk, minced garlic, lemon juice, and fresh mint. Blend until smooth.
2. Heat 1 tablespoon of olive oil in a large skillet over medium-high heat.
3. Add the scallops and cook for 2-3 minutes on each side, until golden brown and cooked through.
4. In a small saucepan, heat the pea puree over low heat until warmed through.
5. Divide the pea puree among four plates. Top with seared scallops.
6. Drizzle with the remaining 1 tablespoon of olive oil before serving.
7. Serve warm.

Nutrition Information (per serving):
- Calories: 250
- Protein: 24g
- Carbohydrates: 18g
- Dietary Fiber: 6g
- Sugars: 6g
- Fat: 10g
- Saturated Fat: 1.5g
- Sodium: 320mg

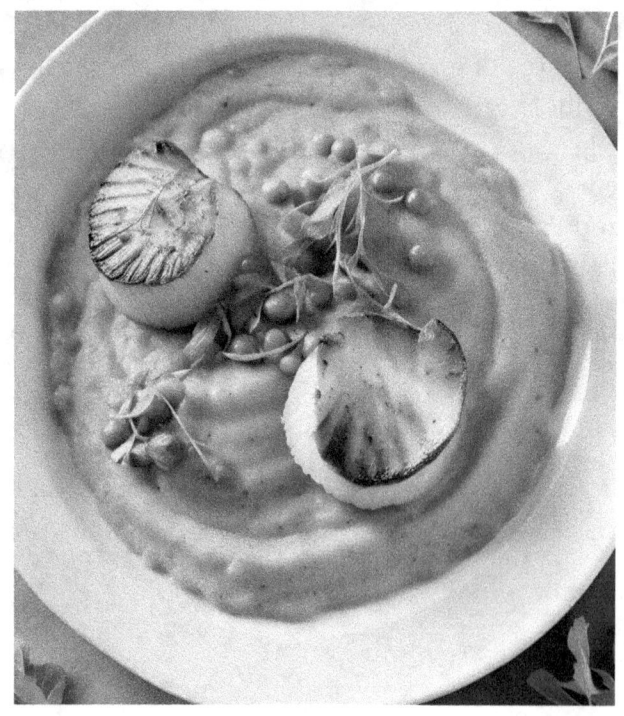

16. Barramundi with Lemon Caper Sauce

Serves: 4
Cooking Time: 25 minutes
Ingredients:
- 4 barramundi fillets (about 6 oz each)
- 2 tablespoons olive oil
- 2 cloves garlic, minced
- 1/4 cup capers, rinsed and drained
- 1/4 cup lemon juice
- 1/4 cup low-sodium chicken broth
- 1 tablespoon fresh parsley, chopped

Instructions:
1. Heat 1 tablespoon of olive oil in a large skillet over medium-high heat.
2. Add the barramundi fillets and cook for 4-5 minutes on each side, until golden brown and cooked through. Remove from skillet and set aside.
3. In the same skillet, add the remaining 1 tablespoon of olive oil and minced garlic. Cook for 1-2 minutes until fragrant.
4. Stir in the capers, lemon juice, and chicken broth. Cook for another 2-3 minutes until the sauce is slightly reduced.
5. Return the barramundi fillets to the skillet, spooning the sauce over the fish. Cook for an additional 2 minutes.
6. Garnish with chopped fresh parsley before serving.
7. Serve warm.

Nutrition Information (per serving):
- Calories: 290
- Protein: 32g
- Carbohydrates: 4g
- Dietary Fiber: 1g
- Sugars: 1g
- Fat: 16g
- Saturated Fat: 2.5g
- Sodium: 360mg

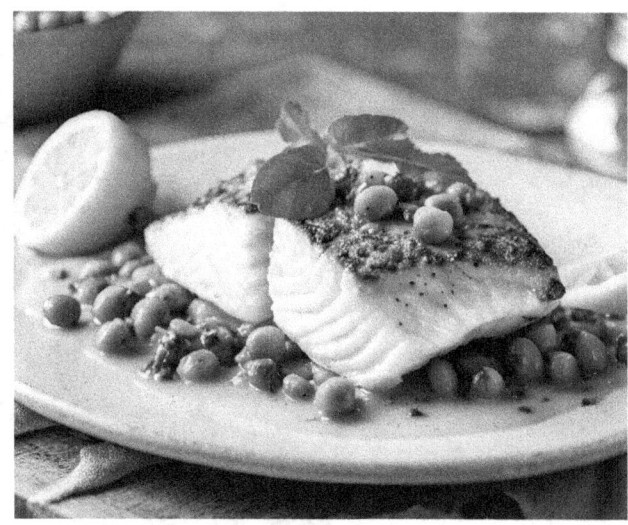

17. Stuffed Trout with Spinach and Pine Nuts

Serves: 4
Cooking Time: 30 minutes
Ingredients:
- 4 whole trout, cleaned and boned
- 2 tablespoons olive oil
- 3 cups fresh spinach, chopped
- 1/4 cup pine nuts, toasted
- 2 cloves garlic, minced
- 1 tablespoon lemon juice
- 1 tablespoon fresh dill, chopped

Instructions:
1. Preheat the oven to 375°F (190°C). Line a baking sheet with parchment paper.
2. In a large skillet, heat 1 tablespoon of olive oil over medium heat. Add the minced garlic and cook for 1-2 minutes until fragrant.
3. Add the chopped spinach and cook until wilted, about 3 minutes. Stir in the toasted pine nuts and lemon juice. Remove from heat.
4. Stuff each trout with the spinach mixture and place on the prepared baking sheet. Drizzle with the remaining 1 tablespoon of olive oil.
5. Bake in the preheated oven for 20-25 minutes, or until the fish is opaque and flakes easily with a fork.
6. Garnish with chopped fresh dill before serving.
7. Serve warm.

Nutrition Information (per serving):
- Calories: 340
- Protein: 32g
- Carbohydrates: 4g
- Dietary Fiber: 2g
- Sugars: 0g
- Fat: 22g
- Saturated Fat: 3g
- Sodium: 150mg

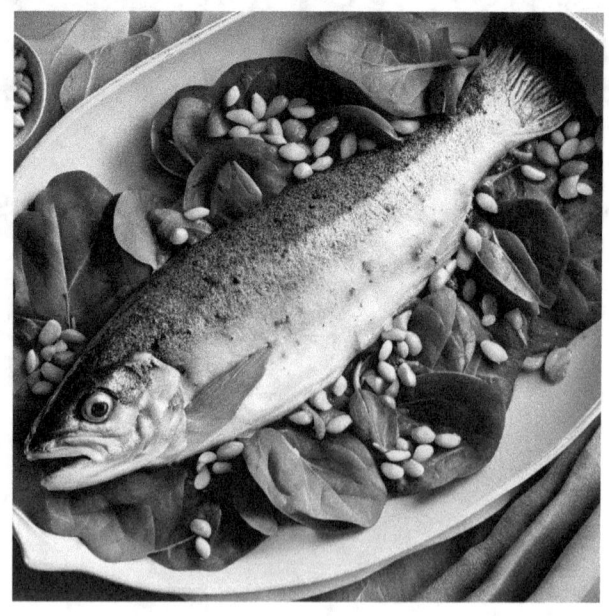

18. Grilled Mackerel with Herb Salad

Serves: 4

Cooking Time: 20 minutes

Ingredients:
- 4 mackerel fillets (about 6 oz each)
- 3 tablespoons olive oil, divided
- 1 tablespoon lemon juice
- 1 teaspoon dried thyme
- 1 cup mixed fresh herbs (parsley, cilantro, mint), chopped
- 1/4 cup red onion, thinly sliced
- 1 cup cherry tomatoes, halved
- 1 tablespoon balsamic vinegar

Instructions:
1. Preheat the grill to medium-high heat.
2. In a small bowl, mix together 2 tablespoons of olive oil, lemon juice, and dried thyme. Brush the mixture over the mackerel fillets.
3. Grill the mackerel fillets for about 5-6 minutes on each side, or until the fish is opaque and flakes easily with a fork.
4. In a large bowl, combine the chopped herbs, sliced red onion, and halved cherry tomatoes.
5. In a small bowl, whisk together the remaining 1 tablespoon of olive oil and balsamic vinegar. Pour over the herb salad and toss to combine.
6. Serve the grilled mackerel fillets topped with the herb salad.
7. Serve warm.

Nutrition Information (per serving):
- Calories: 320
- Protein: 28g
- Carbohydrates: 5g
- Dietary Fiber: 2g
- Sugars: 3g
- Fat: 20g
- Saturated Fat: 4g
- Sodium: 160mg

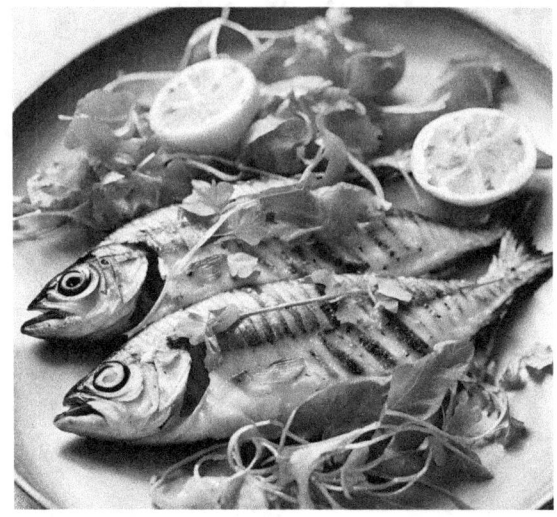

19. Pan-Seared Tuna Steaks

Serves: 4

Cooking Time: 15 minutes

Ingredients:
- 4 tuna steaks (about 6 oz each)
- 2 tablespoons olive oil
- 1 tablespoon lemon juice
- 1 tablespoon low-sodium soy sauce
- 1 teaspoon garlic powder
- 1 teaspoon ground ginger

Instructions:
1. In a small bowl, mix together the olive oil, lemon juice, soy sauce, garlic powder, and ground ginger.
2. Brush the mixture over the tuna steaks, coating them evenly.
3. Heat a large skillet over medium-high heat.
4. Add the tuna steaks and cook for about 2-3 minutes on each side, until seared on the outside but still pink in the center.
5. Remove from heat and let rest for a few minutes before serving.
6. Serve warm.

Nutrition Information (per serving):
- Calories: 280
- Protein: 38g
- Carbohydrates: 1g
- Dietary Fiber: 0g
- Sugars: 0g
- Fat: 14g
- Saturated Fat: 2g
- Sodium: 200mg

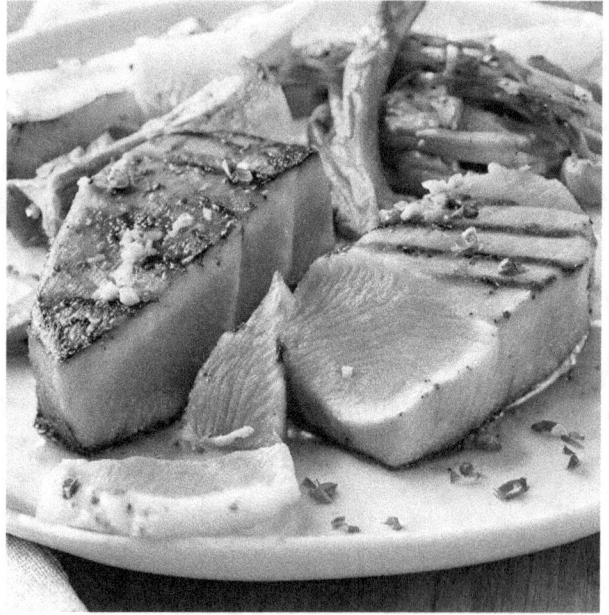

20. Broiled Snapper with Tomato Relish

Serves: 4
Cooking Time: 20 minutes
Ingredients:
- 4 snapper fillets (about 6 oz each)
- 2 tablespoons olive oil
- 1 tablespoon lemon juice
- 1 teaspoon dried oregano
- 1 cup cherry tomatoes, halved
- 1/4 cup red onion, finely chopped
- 1 tablespoon capers, rinsed and drained
- 1 tablespoon fresh basil, chopped
- 1 tablespoon balsamic vinegar

Instructions:
1. Preheat the broiler.
2. In a small bowl, mix together 1 tablespoon of olive oil, lemon juice, and dried oregano.
3. Brush the mixture over the snapper fillets.
4. Place the fillets on a broiler pan and broil for about 6-8 minutes, or until the fish is opaque and flakes easily with a fork.
5. While the fish is broiling, combine the cherry tomatoes, red onion, capers, fresh basil, and balsamic vinegar in a bowl. Toss to combine.
6. Serve the broiled snapper topped with the tomato relish.
7. Serve warm.

Nutrition Information (per serving):
- Calories: 260
- Protein: 30g
- Carbohydrates: 5g
- Dietary Fiber: 1g
- Sugars: 3g
- Fat: 14g
- Saturated Fat: 2g
- Sodium: 240mg

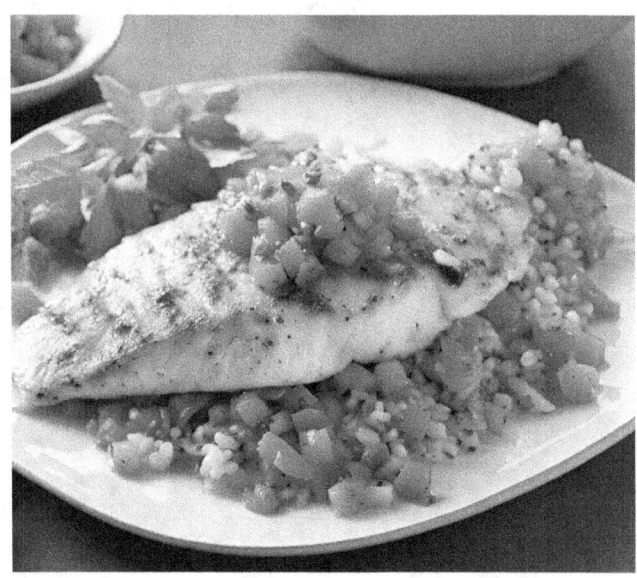

21. Cajun Catfish with Sweet Potato Mash

Serves: 4

Cooking Time: 30 minutes

Ingredients:

For the Catfish:
- 4 catfish fillets (about 6 oz each)
- 2 tablespoons olive oil
- 1 tablespoon Cajun seasoning

For the Sweet Potato Mash:
- 2 large sweet potatoes, peeled and cubed
- 1/4 cup unsweetened almond milk
- 1 tablespoon olive oil
- 1 teaspoon ground cinnamon

Instructions:
1. Preheat the oven to 375°F (190°C).
2. Toss the catfish fillets with olive oil and Cajun seasoning until evenly coated.
3. Place the fillets on a baking sheet and bake for 20-25 minutes, or until the fish is opaque and flakes easily with a fork.
4. While the catfish is baking, bring a large pot of water to a boil. Add the sweet potatoes and cook until tender, about 15 minutes. Drain and return to the pot.
5. Add the almond milk, olive oil, and ground cinnamon to the sweet potatoes. Mash until smooth and well combined.
6. Serve the Cajun catfish with the sweet potato mash.
7. Serve warm.

Nutrition Information (per serving):
- Calories: 350
- Protein: 28g
- Carbohydrates: 30g
- Dietary Fiber: 5g
- Sugars: 8g
- Fat: 16g
- Saturated Fat: 2.5g
- Sodium: 320mg

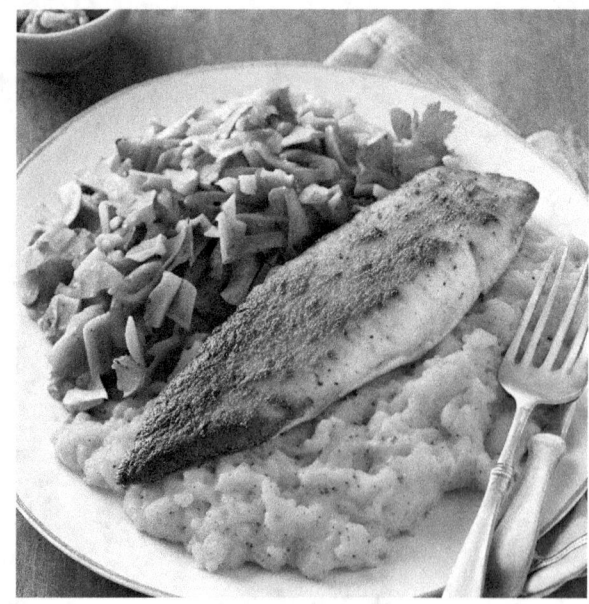

22. Shrimp and Asparagus Stir-fry

Serves: 4
Cooking Time: 15 minutes
Ingredients:

- 1 pound large shrimp, peeled and deveined
- 2 tablespoons olive oil
- 2 cloves garlic, minced
- 1 tablespoon fresh ginger, minced
- 1 bunch asparagus, trimmed and cut into 2-inch pieces
- 1 red bell pepper, sliced
- 3 tablespoons low-sodium soy sauce
- 1 tablespoon rice vinegar
- 1 tablespoon honey or maple syrup (optional)

Instructions:

1. Heat 1 tablespoon of olive oil in a large skillet or wok over medium-high heat.
2. Add the shrimp and cook for about 2-3 minutes on each side, until pink and cooked through. Remove from the skillet and set aside.
3. Add the remaining 1 tablespoon of olive oil to the skillet. Add the minced garlic and ginger, cooking for 1-2 minutes until fragrant.
4. Add the asparagus and red bell pepper, stir-frying for about 5-7 minutes, until the vegetables are tender-crisp.
5. Return the shrimp to the skillet.
6. In a small bowl, mix together the soy sauce, rice vinegar, and honey or maple syrup (if using). Pour the sauce over the shrimp and vegetables, stirring to combine.
7. Cook for another 2-3 minutes, until everything is heated through.
8. Serve warm.

Nutrition Information (per serving):

- Calories: 250
- Protein: 24g
- Carbohydrates: 12g
- Dietary Fiber: 3g
- Sugars: 5g
- Fat: 12g
- Saturated Fat: 2g
- Sodium: 420mg

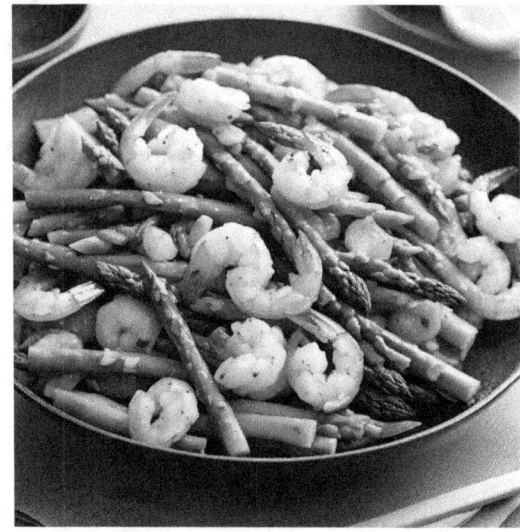

23. Mediterranean Baked Sardines

Serves: 4
Cooking Time: 25 minutes

Ingredients:
- 8 fresh sardines, cleaned
- 3 tablespoons olive oil
- 1 lemon, thinly sliced
- 1/4 cup Kalamata olives, pitted and sliced
- 2 cloves garlic, minced
- 1 tablespoon fresh oregano, chopped
- 1 tablespoon fresh parsley, chopped

Instructions:
1. Preheat the oven to 375°F (190°C). Line a baking dish with parchment paper.
2. In a small bowl, mix together the olive oil, minced garlic, chopped oregano, and chopped parsley.
3. Arrange the sardines in the prepared baking dish. Drizzle with the olive oil mixture.
4. Top with lemon slices and Kalamata olives.
5. Bake in the preheated oven for 15-20 minutes, or until the sardines are cooked through and the flesh flakes easily with a fork.
6. Serve warm.

Nutrition Information (per serving):
- Calories: 220
- Protein: 20g
- Carbohydrates: 2g
- Dietary Fiber: 0g
- Sugars: 0g
- Fat: 15g
- Saturated Fat: 2.5g
- Sodium: 300mg

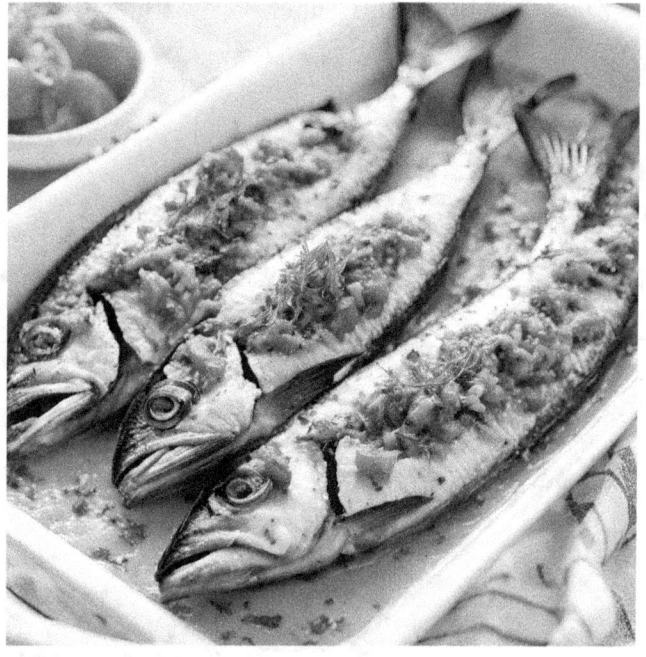

24. Flounder with Parsley Sauce

Serves: 4
Cooking Time: 20 minutes
Ingredients:
- 4 flounder fillets (about 6 oz each)
- 2 tablespoons olive oil
- 1 cup fresh parsley, chopped
- 2 cloves garlic, minced
- 1 tablespoon lemon juice
- 1/4 cup low-sodium chicken broth

Instructions:
1. Preheat the oven to 375°F (190°C). Line a baking dish with parchment paper.
2. Place the flounder fillets in the prepared baking dish. Drizzle with olive oil.
3. In a small bowl, mix together the chopped parsley, minced garlic, lemon juice, and chicken broth.
4. Pour the parsley sauce over the flounder fillets.
5. Bake in the preheated oven for 15-20 minutes, or until the fish is opaque and flakes easily with a fork.
6. Serve warm.

Nutrition Information (per serving):
- Calories: 220
- Protein: 30g
- Carbohydrates: 2g
- Dietary Fiber: 0g
- Sugars: 0g
- Fat: 10g
- Saturated Fat: 1.5g
- Sodium: 120mg

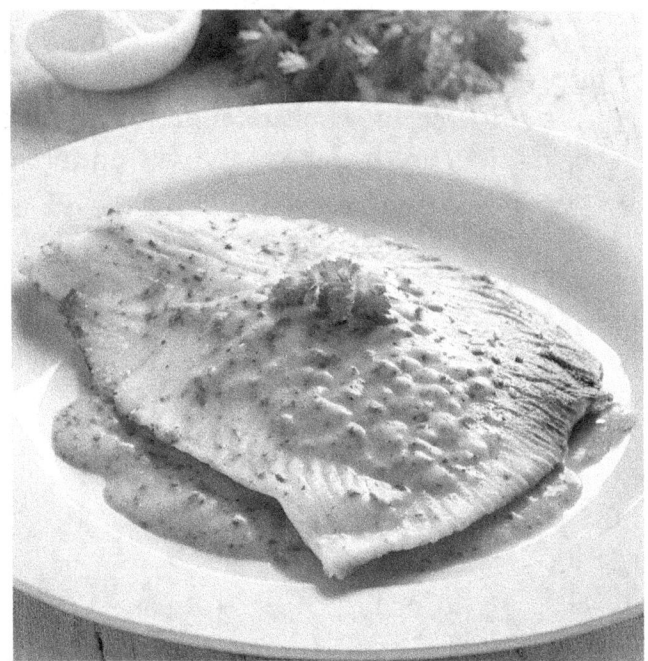

25. Scallop and Chorizo Paella

Serves: 4
Cooking Time: 40 minutes

Ingredients:
- 1 tablespoon olive oil
- 1/2 pound chorizo, sliced
- 1 pound sea scallops
- 1 onion, diced
- 2 cloves garlic, minced
- 1 red bell pepper, diced
- 1 cup Arborio rice
- 2 cups low-sodium chicken broth
- 1/4 teaspoon saffron threads (optional)
- 1 cup frozen peas, thawed
- 1 tablespoon lemon juice
- 1/4 cup fresh parsley, chopped

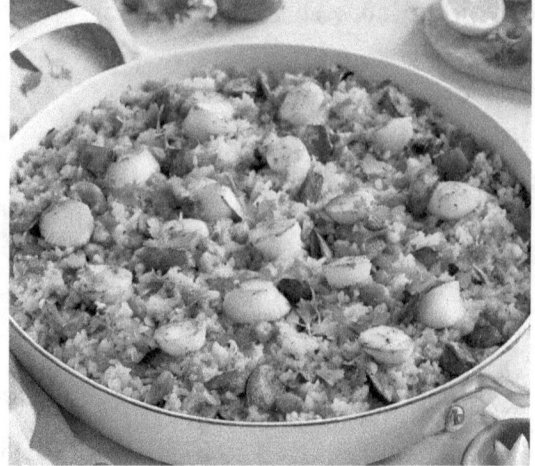

Instructions:
1. Heat olive oil in a large skillet or paella pan over medium heat. Add the sliced chorizo and cook for about 5 minutes until browned. Remove from the skillet and set aside.
2. Add the sea scallops to the skillet and cook for about 2-3 minutes on each side until browned. Remove from the skillet and set aside.
3. Add the diced onion, minced garlic, and red bell pepper to the skillet. Cook for about 5 minutes until softened.
4. Stir in the Arborio rice and cook for about 2 minutes until lightly toasted.
5. Pour in the chicken broth and add the saffron threads (if using). Bring to a boil, then reduce heat to low and simmer for about 20 minutes until the rice is cooked and the liquid is absorbed.
6. Stir in the cooked chorizo, thawed peas, and lemon juice. Cook for an additional 5 minutes.
7. Return the cooked scallops to the skillet and cook for about 2 minutes until heated through.
8. Garnish with chopped fresh parsley before serving.
9. Serve warm.

Nutrition Information (per serving):
- Calories: 400
- Protein: 30g
- Carbohydrates: 40g
- Dietary Fiber: 5g
- Sugars: 3g
- Fat: 15g
- Saturated Fat: 5g
- Sodium: 480mg

26. Anchovy and Green Bean Salad

Serves: 4
Cooking Time: 15 minutes
Ingredients:
- 1 pound fresh green beans, trimmed
- 1/4 cup olive oil
- 1 tablespoon lemon juice
- 2 cloves garlic, minced
- 1/4 cup sliced almonds, toasted
- 1 can (2 oz) anchovy fillets, drained and chopped
- 1/4 cup fresh parsley, chopped

Instructions:
1. Bring a large pot of water to a boil. Add the green beans and cook for about 5 minutes until tender-crisp. Drain and rinse under cold water to stop the cooking process.
2. In a small bowl, whisk together the olive oil, lemon juice, and minced garlic.
3. In a large bowl, combine the cooked green beans, toasted almonds, chopped anchovies, and fresh parsley.
4. Pour the dressing over the salad and toss to combine.
5. Serve immediately.

Nutrition Information (per serving):
- Calories: 220
- Protein: 6g
- Carbohydrates: 8g
- Dietary Fiber: 4g
- Sugars: 2g
- Fat: 18g
- Saturated Fat: 2.5g
- Sodium: 320mg

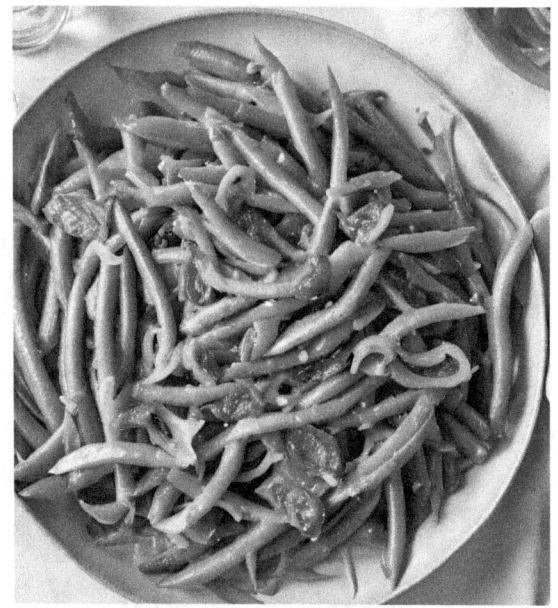

27. Honey Glazed Salmon

Serves: 4
Cooking Time: 20 minutes
Ingredients:
- 4 salmon fillets (about 6 oz each)
- 2 tablespoons olive oil
- 1/4 cup honey
- 2 tablespoons lemon juice
- 2 cloves garlic, minced
- 1 teaspoon ground ginger
- 1 tablespoon fresh thyme leaves

Instructions:
1. Preheat the oven to 375°F (190°C). Line a baking dish with parchment paper.
2. In a small bowl, whisk together the honey, lemon juice, minced garlic, ground ginger, and fresh thyme leaves.
3. Place the salmon fillets in the prepared baking dish. Drizzle with olive oil.
4. Pour the honey glaze over the salmon fillets.
5. Bake in the preheated oven for 15-20 minutes, or until the salmon is cooked through and flakes easily with a fork.
6. Serve warm.

Nutrition Information (per serving):
- Calories: 360
- Protein: 34g
- Carbohydrates: 18g
- Dietary Fiber: 0g
- Sugars: 16g
- Fat: 16g
- Saturated Fat: 3g
- Sodium: 80mg

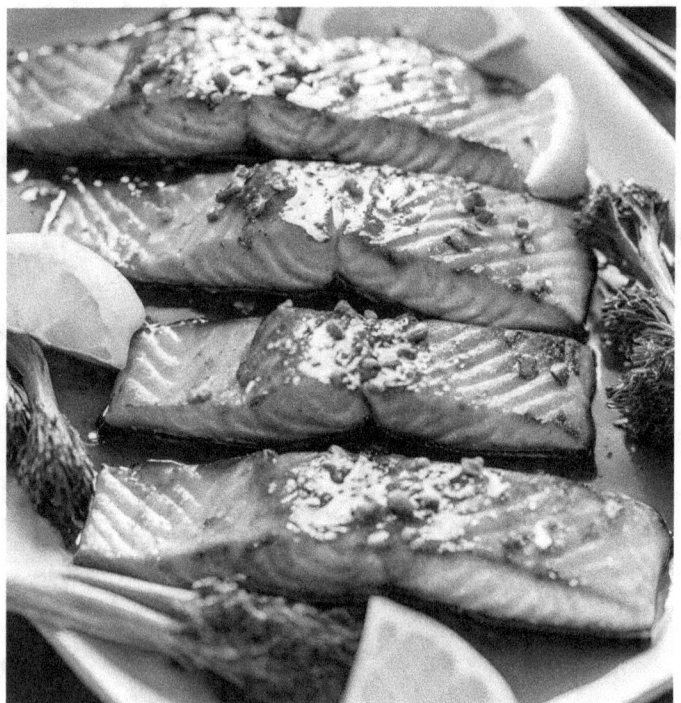

Soup & Stew Recipes

1. Lentil and Spinach Soup
Serves: 6
Cooking Time: 40 minutes
Ingredients:
- 2 tablespoons olive oil
- 1 large onion, diced
- 3 cloves garlic, minced
- 2 carrots, diced
- 2 celery stalks, diced
- 1 cup dried lentils, rinsed
- 6 cups low-sodium vegetable broth
- 1 teaspoon ground cumin
- 1 teaspoon ground coriander
- 1 teaspoon paprika
- 4 cups fresh spinach, chopped
- 1 tablespoon lemon juice

Instructions:
1. In a large pot, heat the olive oil over medium heat. Add the diced onion and garlic, cooking until softened, about 5 minutes.
2. Add the diced carrots and celery, cooking for another 5 minutes.
3. Stir in the lentils, vegetable broth, ground cumin, ground coriander, and paprika. Bring to a boil, then reduce heat and simmer for 25-30 minutes, or until the lentils are tender.
4. Stir in the chopped spinach and cook for an additional 5 minutes, until wilted.
5. Stir in the lemon juice before serving.
6. Serve warm.

Nutrition Information (per serving):
- Calories: 180
- Protein: 8g
- Carbohydrates: 28g
- Dietary Fiber: 8g
- Sugars: 4g
- Fat: 5g
- Saturated Fat: 0.5g
- Sodium: 260mg

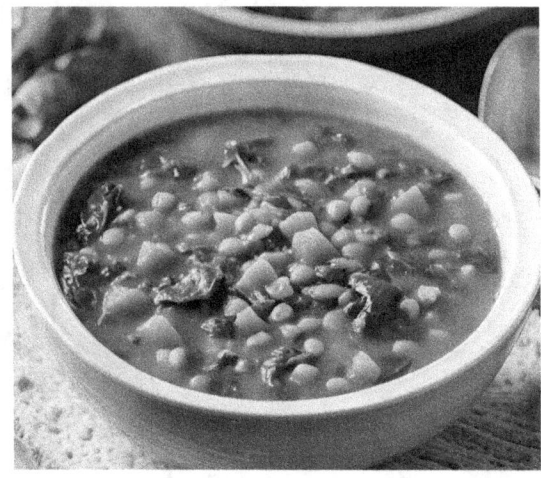

2. Split Pea Soup

Serves: 6
Cooking Time: 1 hour
Ingredients:

- 2 tablespoons olive oil
- 1 large onion, diced
- 3 cloves garlic, minced
- 2 carrots, diced
- 2 celery stalks, diced
- 2 cups dried split peas, rinsed
- 8 cups low-sodium vegetable broth
- 1 teaspoon dried thyme
- 1 teaspoon dried oregano
- 1 bay leaf
- 1 tablespoon apple cider vinegar

Instructions:

1. In a large pot, heat the olive oil over medium heat. Add the diced onion and garlic, cooking until softened, about 5 minutes.
2. Add the diced carrots and celery, cooking for another 5 minutes.
3. Stir in the split peas, vegetable broth, dried thyme, dried oregano, and bay leaf. Bring to a boil, then reduce heat and simmer for 45-50 minutes, or until the peas are tender.
4. Remove the bay leaf and stir in the apple cider vinegar.
5. Serve warm.

Nutrition Information (per serving):

- Calories: 220
- Protein: 13g
- Carbohydrates: 38g
- Dietary Fiber: 14g
- Sugars: 7g
- Fat: 4g
- Saturated Fat: 0.5g
- Sodium: 300mg

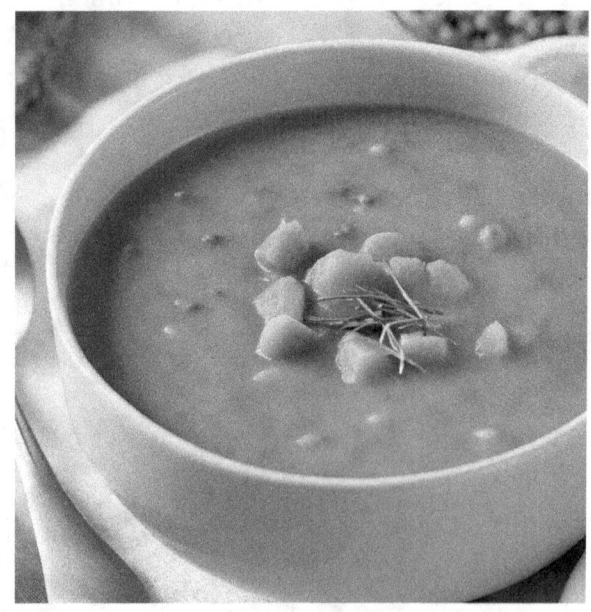

3. White Bean and Kale Soup

Serves: 6
Cooking Time: 35 minutes
Ingredients:
- 2 tablespoons olive oil
- 1 large onion, diced
- 3 cloves garlic, minced
- 2 carrots, diced
- 2 celery stalks, diced
- 4 cups kale, chopped
- 2 cans (15 oz each) white beans, drained and rinsed
- 6 cups low-sodium vegetable broth
- 1 teaspoon dried thyme
- 1 teaspoon dried basil
- 1 tablespoon lemon juice

Instructions:
1. In a large pot, heat the olive oil over medium heat. Add the diced onion and garlic, cooking until softened, about 5 minutes.
2. Add the diced carrots and celery, cooking for another 5 minutes.
3. Stir in the chopped kale and cook until wilted, about 3 minutes.
4. Add the white beans, vegetable broth, dried thyme, and dried basil. Bring to a boil, then reduce heat and simmer for 20 minutes.
5. Stir in the lemon juice before serving.
6. Serve warm.

Nutrition Information (per serving):
- Calories: 190
- Protein: 10g
- Carbohydrates: 30g
- Dietary Fiber: 10g
- Sugars: 4g
- Fat: 5g
- Saturated Fat: 0.5g
- Sodium: 300mg

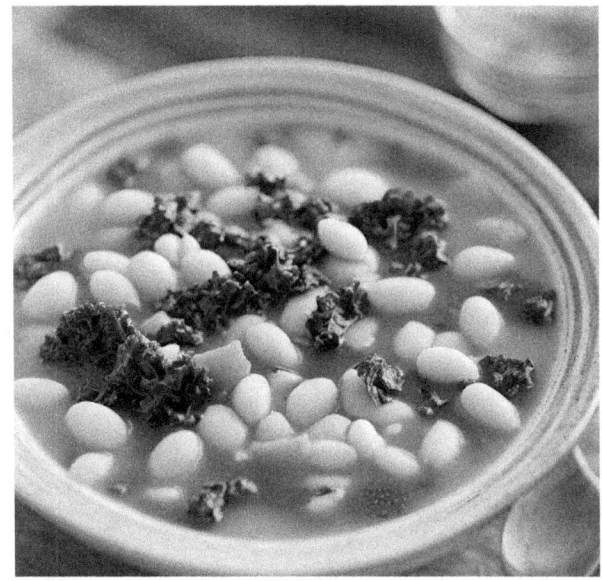

4. Thai Coconut Shrimp Soup

Serves: 4
Cooking Time: 25 minutes
Ingredients:
- 2 tablespoons olive oil
- 1 onion, diced
- 3 cloves garlic, minced
- 1 tablespoon fresh ginger, minced
- 1 red bell pepper, sliced
- 1 pound large shrimp, peeled and deveined
- 1 can (14 oz) coconut milk
- 4 cups low-sodium chicken broth
- 2 tablespoons fish sauce
- 1 tablespoon red curry paste
- 1 tablespoon lime juice
- 1/4 cup fresh cilantro, chopped

Instructions:
1. In a large pot, heat the olive oil over medium heat. Add the diced onion, minced garlic, and fresh ginger, cooking until softened, about 5 minutes.
2. Add the sliced red bell pepper and cook for another 5 minutes.
3. Stir in the shrimp and cook until pink, about 3-4 minutes.
4. Add the coconut milk, chicken broth, fish sauce, and red curry paste. Bring to a simmer and cook for 10 minutes.
5. Stir in the lime juice and chopped fresh cilantro.
6. Serve warm.

Nutrition Information (per serving):
- Calories: 320
- Protein: 24g
- Carbohydrates: 12g
- Dietary Fiber: 2g
- Sugars: 5g
- Fat: 22g
- Saturated Fat: 16g
- Sodium: 600mg

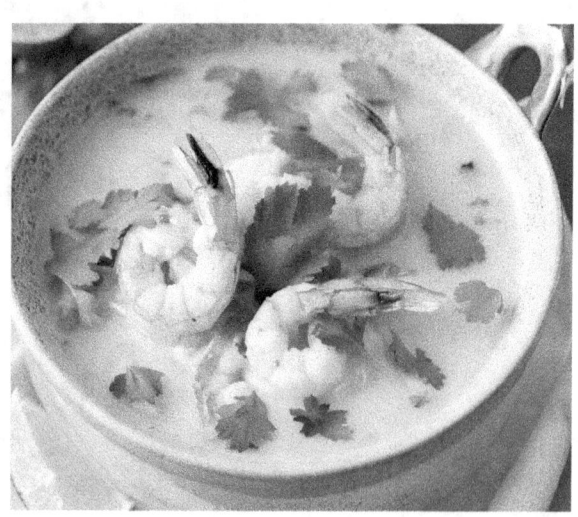

5. Miso Soup with Tofu

Serves: 4
Cooking Time: 15 minutes
Ingredients:

- 4 cups water
- 1/4 cup miso paste
- 1 cup silken tofu, cubed
- 1 cup wakame seaweed, rehydrated
- 2 green onions, sliced
- 1 tablespoon low-sodium soy sauce

Instructions:

1. In a large pot, bring the water to a boil. Reduce heat to low and stir in the miso paste until dissolved.
2. Add the cubed tofu and rehydrated wakame seaweed. Simmer for about 5 minutes.
3. Stir in the sliced green onions and soy sauce.
4. Serve warm.

Nutrition Information (per serving):

- Calories: 80
- Protein: 5g
- Carbohydrates: 7g
- Dietary Fiber: 1g
- Sugars: 2g
- Fat: 3g
- Saturated Fat: 0.5g
- Sodium: 400mg

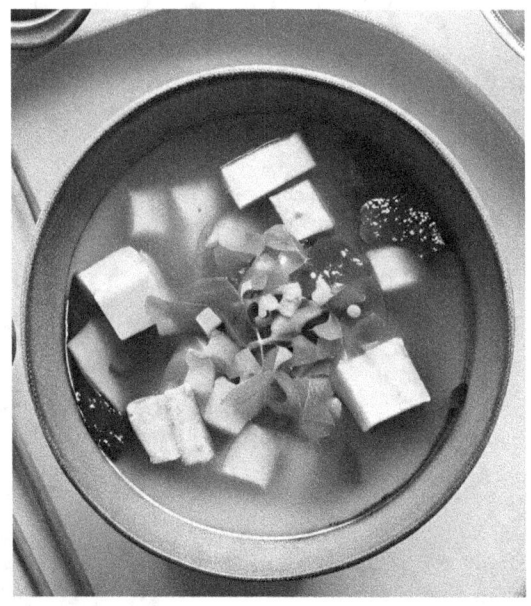

6. Vegetable Beef Stew

Serves: 6
Cooking Time: 2 hours
Ingredients:
- 2 tablespoons olive oil
- 1 pound beef stew meat, cubed
- 1 large onion, diced
- 3 cloves garlic, minced
- 4 carrots, diced
- 3 celery stalks, diced
- 3 potatoes, peeled and cubed
- 1 cup green beans, trimmed and cut into 1-inch pieces
- 1 cup peas
- 6 cups low-sodium beef broth
- 1 teaspoon dried thyme
- 1 teaspoon dried rosemary
- 2 tablespoons tomato paste
- 1 tablespoon Worcestershire sauce

Instructions:
1. In a large pot, heat the olive oil over medium-high heat. Add the beef stew meat and cook until browned on all sides. Remove the meat from the pot and set aside.
2. In the same pot, add the diced onion and garlic, cooking until softened, about 5 minutes.
3. Add the carrots, celery, and potatoes, cooking for another 5 minutes.
4. Stir in the beef broth, dried thyme, dried rosemary, tomato paste, and Worcestershire sauce. Return the browned beef to the pot.
5. Bring the mixture to a boil, then reduce heat to low and simmer for 1.5 hours.
6. Add the green beans and peas, cooking for an additional 20 minutes, until the vegetables are tender.
7. Serve warm.

Nutrition Information (per serving):
- Calories: 280
- Protein: 22g
- Carbohydrates: 30g
- Dietary Fiber: 6g
- Sugars: 7g
- Fat: 10g
- Saturated Fat: 2.5g
- Sodium: 420mg

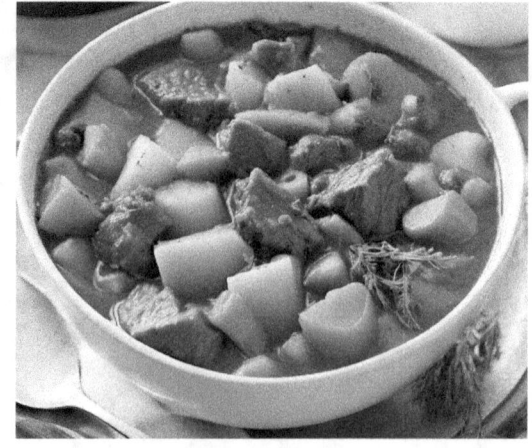

7. Chicken Tortilla Soup

Serves: 6
Cooking Time: 40 minutes
Ingredients:

- 2 tablespoons olive oil
- 1 large onion, diced
- 3 cloves garlic, minced
- 1 jalapeño, seeded and diced
- 1 red bell pepper, diced
- 1 can (14.5 oz) diced tomatoes
- 6 cups low-sodium chicken broth
- 1 teaspoon ground cumin
- 1 teaspoon chili powder
- 2 cups cooked shredded chicken
- 1 cup corn kernels (fresh or frozen)
- 1 cup black beans, rinsed and drained
- 1/4 cup fresh cilantro, chopped
- 1 tablespoon lime juice
- 6 small whole wheat tortillas, cut into strips

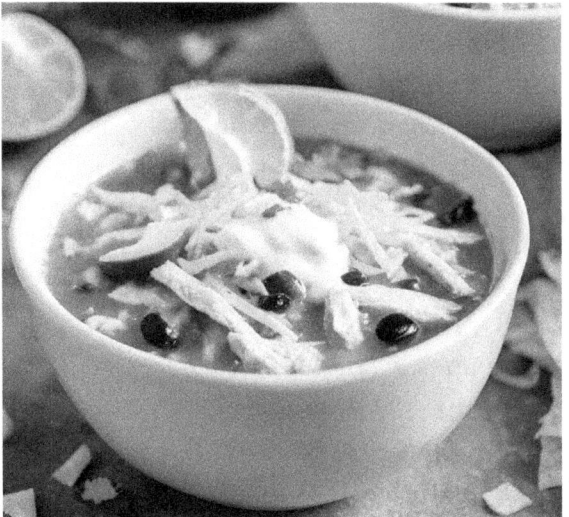

Instructions:

1. In a large pot, heat the olive oil over medium heat. Add the diced onion, garlic, jalapeño, and red bell pepper, cooking until softened, about 5 minutes.
2. Stir in the diced tomatoes, chicken broth, ground cumin, and chili powder. Bring to a boil.
3. Reduce heat to low and simmer for 15 minutes.
4. Add the shredded chicken, corn kernels, and black beans. Simmer for an additional 10 minutes.
5. Stir in the chopped cilantro and lime juice.
6. Serve the soup topped with tortilla strips.
7. Serve warm.

Nutrition Information (per serving):

- Calories: 300
- Protein: 22g
- Carbohydrates: 38g
- Dietary Fiber: 8g
- Sugars: 6g
- Fat: 10g
- Saturated Fat: 1.5g
- Sodium: 480mg

8. Barley and Mushroom Soup

Serves: 6
Cooking Time: 1 hour
Ingredients:
- 2 tablespoons olive oil
- 1 large onion, diced
- 3 cloves garlic, minced
- 3 carrots, diced
- 2 celery stalks, diced
- 8 oz mushrooms, sliced
- 1 cup pearl barley
- 6 cups low-sodium vegetable broth
- 1 teaspoon dried thyme
- 1 teaspoon dried sage
- 1 tablespoon soy sauce
- 1/4 cup fresh parsley, chopped

Instructions:
1. In a large pot, heat the olive oil over medium heat. Add the diced onion and garlic, cooking until softened, about 5 minutes.
2. Add the carrots, celery, and mushrooms, cooking for another 5 minutes.
3. Stir in the pearl barley, vegetable broth, dried thyme, dried sage, and soy sauce. Bring to a boil.
4. Reduce heat to low and simmer for 45 minutes, or until the barley is tender.
5. Stir in the chopped fresh parsley before serving.
6. Serve warm.

Nutrition Information (per serving):
- Calories: 230
- Protein: 6g
- Carbohydrates: 40g
- Dietary Fiber: 8g
- Sugars: 7g
- Fat: 7g
- Saturated Fat: 1g
- Sodium: 350mg

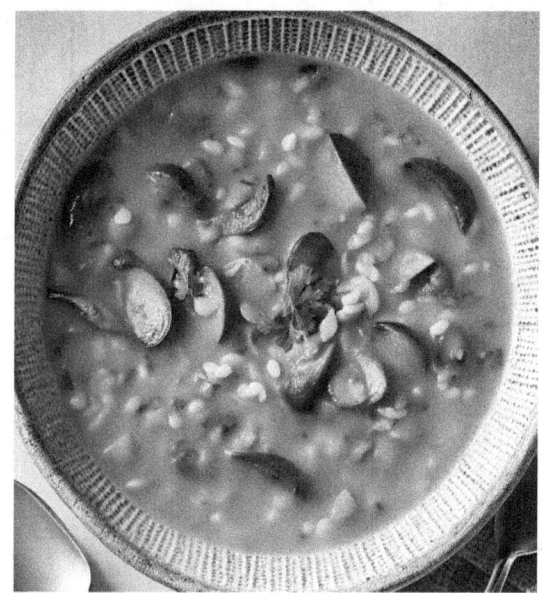

9. Spicy Black Bean Soup

Serves: 6
Cooking Time: 40 minutes

Ingredients:
- 2 tablespoons olive oil
- 1 large onion, diced
- 3 cloves garlic, minced
- 1 jalapeño, seeded and diced
- 1 red bell pepper, diced
- 2 cans (15 oz each) black beans, rinsed and drained
- 4 cups low-sodium vegetable broth
- 1 teaspoon ground cumin
- 1 teaspoon chili powder
- 1 teaspoon smoked paprika
- 1 tablespoon lime juice
- 1/4 cup fresh cilantro, chopped

Instructions:
1. In a large pot, heat the olive oil over medium heat. Add the diced onion, garlic, jalapeño, and red bell pepper, cooking until softened, about 5 minutes.
2. Stir in the black beans, vegetable broth, ground cumin, chili powder, and smoked paprika. Bring to a boil.
3. Reduce heat to low and simmer for 25 minutes.
4. Using an immersion blender, blend the soup until smooth, or to your desired consistency.
5. Stir in the lime juice and chopped fresh cilantro.
6. Serve warm.

Nutrition Information (per serving):
- Calories: 200
- Protein: 8g
- Carbohydrates: 30g
- Dietary Fiber: 10g
- Sugars: 5g
- Fat: 7g
- Saturated Fat: 1g
- Sodium: 320mg

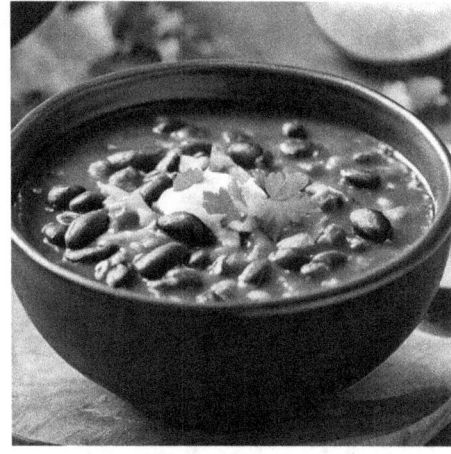

10. Italian Sausage and Potato Soup

Serves: 6
Cooking Time: 45 minutes
Ingredients:
- 1 pound Italian sausage (preferably turkey or chicken sausage)
- 2 tablespoons olive oil
- 1 large onion, diced
- 3 cloves garlic, minced
- 4 cups potatoes, peeled and diced
- 4 cups low-sodium chicken broth
- 2 cups kale, chopped
- 1 teaspoon dried oregano
- 1 teaspoon dried basil
- 1/2 cup unsweetened almond milk

Instructions:
1. In a large pot, cook the Italian sausage over medium heat until browned. Remove the sausage from the pot and set aside.
2. In the same pot, add the olive oil, diced onion, and garlic. Cook until the onion is softened, about 5 minutes.
3. Add the diced potatoes, chicken broth, dried oregano, and dried basil. Bring to a boil, then reduce heat and simmer for 20-25 minutes, or until the potatoes are tender.
4. Stir in the cooked sausage, chopped kale, and almond milk. Simmer for an additional 5-10 minutes, until the kale is wilted and the soup is heated through.
5. Serve warm.

Nutrition Information (per serving):
- Calories: 300
- Protein: 18g
- Carbohydrates: 30g
- Dietary Fiber: 5g
- Sugars: 3g
- Fat: 14g
- Saturated Fat: 3.5g
- Sodium: 450mg

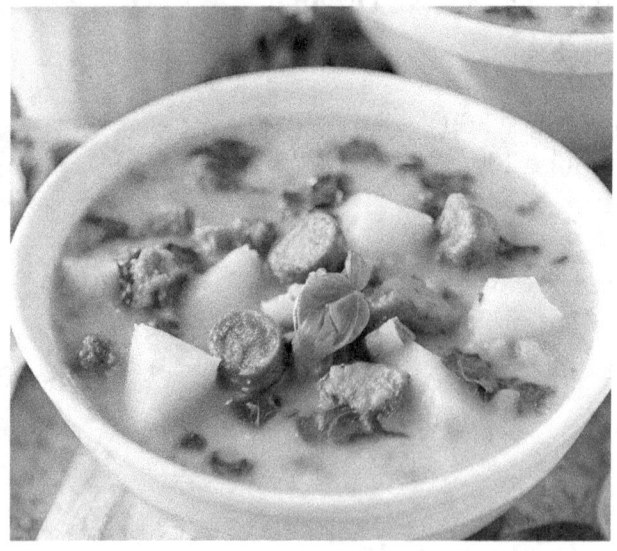

11. Sweet Potato and Red Lentil Soup

Serves: 6
Cooking Time: 45 minutes
Ingredients:
- 2 tablespoons olive oil
- 1 large onion, diced
- 3 cloves garlic, minced
- 2 large sweet potatoes, peeled and diced
- 1 cup red lentils, rinsed
- 6 cups low-sodium vegetable broth
- 1 teaspoon ground cumin
- 1 teaspoon ground coriander
- 1 teaspoon smoked paprika
- 1 tablespoon lemon juice
- 1/4 cup fresh cilantro, chopped

Instructions:
1. In a large pot, heat the olive oil over medium heat. Add the diced onion and garlic, cooking until softened, about 5 minutes.
2. Add the diced sweet potatoes, red lentils, vegetable broth, ground cumin, ground coriander, and smoked paprika. Bring to a boil.
3. Reduce heat and simmer for 30-35 minutes, or until the sweet potatoes and lentils are tender.
4. Using an immersion blender, blend the soup until smooth, or to your desired consistency.
5. Stir in the lemon juice and chopped fresh cilantro.
6. Serve warm.

Nutrition Information (per serving):
- Calories: 220
- Protein: 7g
- Carbohydrates: 36g
- Dietary Fiber: 10g
- Sugars: 8g
- Fat: 6g
- Saturated Fat: 1g
- Sodium: 320mg

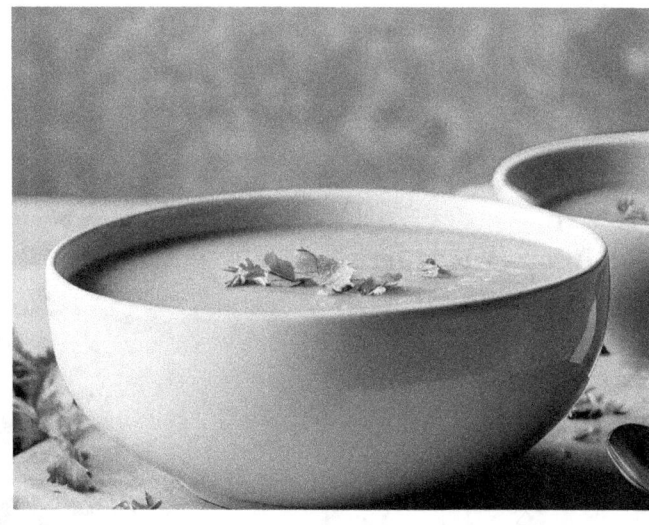

12. Caribbean Chicken Stew

Serves: 6
Cooking Time: 1 hour
Ingredients:
- 2 tablespoons olive oil
- 1 pound boneless, skinless chicken thighs, cut into bite-sized pieces
- 1 large onion, diced
- 3 cloves garlic, minced
- 1 red bell pepper, diced
- 1 green bell pepper, diced
- 2 cups sweet potatoes, peeled and diced
- 1 can (14.5 oz) diced tomatoes
- 4 cups low-sodium chicken broth
- 1 teaspoon ground allspice
- 1 teaspoon dried thyme
- 1/2 teaspoon ground cinnamon
- 1/2 teaspoon ground ginger
- 1 tablespoon apple cider vinegar
- 1/4 cup fresh parsley, chopped

Instructions:
1. In a large pot, heat the olive oil over medium heat. Add the chicken pieces and cook until browned, about 5-7 minutes. Remove the chicken from the pot and set aside.
2. In the same pot, add the diced onion and garlic. Cook until the onion is softened, about 5 minutes.
3. Add the red and green bell peppers, and cook for another 5 minutes.
4. Stir in the sweet potatoes, diced tomatoes, chicken broth, ground allspice, dried thyme, ground cinnamon, and ground ginger. Bring to a boil.
5. Reduce heat and simmer for 30 minutes, or until the sweet potatoes are tender.
6. Return the chicken to the pot and stir in the apple cider vinegar. Simmer for an additional 10 minutes, until the chicken is cooked through and the flavors are well combined.
7. Garnish with chopped fresh parsley before serving.
8. Serve warm.

Nutrition Information (per serving):
- Calories: 280
- Protein: 20g
- Carbohydrates: 28g
- Dietary Fiber: 6g
- Sugars: 9g
- Fat: 10g
- Saturated Fat: 2g
- Sodium: 380mg

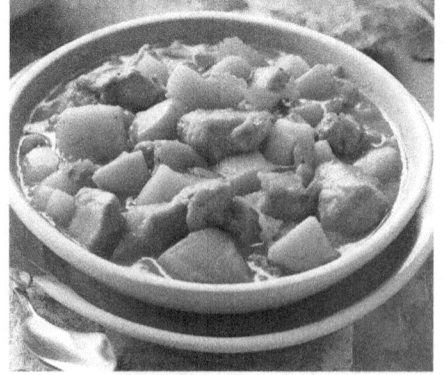

10-WEEK MEAL PLAN

Week 1
Day 1:
- Breakfast: Oatmeal with Walnuts
- Lunch: Lentil and Spinach Soup
- Dinner: Grilled Salmon with Lemon and Herbs

Day 2:
- Breakfast: Spinach and Mushroom Omelette
- Lunch: Split Pea Soup
- Dinner: Herb-Crusted Tilapia

Day 3:
- Breakfast: Greek Yogurt Parfait
- Lunch: White Bean and Kale Soup
- Dinner: Baked Cod with Olive Tapenade

Day 4:
- Breakfast: Almond Flour Pancakes
- Lunch: Vegetable Beef Stew
- Dinner: Pan-Seared Tuna Steaks

Day 5:
- Breakfast: Buckwheat Porridge
- Lunch: Chicken Tortilla Soup
- Dinner: Sardines in Tomato Sauce

Day 6:
- Breakfast: Turkey Sausage Scramble
- Lunch: Barley and Mushroom Soup
- Dinner: Thai Coconut Shrimp Soup

Day 7:
- Breakfast: Quinoa Breakfast Bowl
- Lunch: Spicy Black Bean Soup
- Dinner: Mediterranean Baked Sardines

Week 2
Day 1:
- Breakfast: Kale and Tomato Frittata
- Lunch: Italian Sausage and Potato Soup
- Dinner: Roasted Turkey Breast

Day 2:
- Breakfast: Vegan Tofu Scramble
- Lunch: Sweet Potato and Red Lentil Soup
- Dinner: Chicken Bruschetta

Day 3:
- Breakfast: Sweet Potato Hash
- Lunch: Caribbean Chicken Stew
- Dinner: Asian-Inspired Tuna Poke Bowl

Day 4:
- Breakfast: Pumpkin Oatmeal
- Lunch: Lentil and Spinach Soup
- Dinner: Lemon Butter Haddock

Day 5:
- Breakfast: Millet Porridge
- Lunch: Split Pea Soup
- Dinner: Scallops with Pea Puree

Day 6:
- Breakfast: Egg Muffins
- Lunch: White Bean and Kale Soup
- Dinner: Barramundi with Lemon Caper Sauce

Day 7:
- Breakfast: Zucchini Bread
- Lunch: Vegetable Beef Stew
- Dinner: Stuffed Trout with Spinach and Pine Nuts

Week 3

Day 1:
- Breakfast: Savory Quinoa Bowl
- Lunch: Chicken Tortilla Soup
- Dinner: Grilled Mackerel with Herb Salad

Day 2:
- Breakfast: Kefir with Berries
- Lunch: Barley and Mushroom Soup
- Dinner: Turkey and Cabbage Stir-fry

Day 3:
- Breakfast: Almond Butter Smoothie
- Lunch: Spicy Black Bean Soup
- Dinner: Balsamic Glazed Chicken Breast

Day 4:
- Breakfast: Bircher Muesli
- Lunch: Italian Sausage and Potato Soup
- Dinner: Pesto Turkey Pinwheels

Day 5:
- Breakfast: Turkey and Spinach Crepes
- Lunch: Sweet Potato and Red Lentil Soup
- Dinner: Roasted Chicken with Root Vegetables

Day 6:
- Breakfast: Berry and Chia Yogurt
- Lunch: Caribbean Chicken Stew
- Dinner: Flounder with Parsley Sauce

Day 7:
- Breakfast: Flaxseed and Banana Muffins
- Lunch: Lentil and Spinach Soup
- Dinner: Scallop and Chorizo Paella

Week 4

Day 1:
- Breakfast: Lentil Salad with Poached Eggs
- Lunch: Split Pea Soup
- Dinner: Anchovy and Green Bean Salad

Day 2:
- Breakfast: Baked Cod with Olives and Tomatoes
- Lunch: White Bean and Kale Soup
- Dinner: Honey Glazed Salmon

Day 3:
- Breakfast: Roasted Brussels Sprouts with Garlic
- Lunch: Vegetable Beef Stew
- Dinner: Chicken and Asparagus Stir-fry

Day 4:
- Breakfast: Kale and Quinoa Salad
- Lunch: Chicken Tortilla Soup
- Dinner: Turkey Meatballs in Marinara Sauce

Day 5:
- Breakfast: Zucchini Noodles with Pesto
- Lunch: Barley and Mushroom Soup
- Dinner: Roasted Turnips with Parsley

Day 6:
- Breakfast: Butternut Squash Risotto
- Lunch: Spicy Black Bean Soup
- Dinner: Chicken and Vegetable Kebabs

Day 7:
- Breakfast: Spinach and Feta Stuffed Mushrooms
- Lunch: Italian Sausage and Potato Soup
- Dinner: Buffalo Chicken Salad

Week 5

Day 1:
- Breakfast: Grilled Eggplant with Tomato and Basil
- Lunch: Sweet Potato and Red Lentil Soup
- Dinner: Herb-Roasted Turkey Legs

Day 2:
- Breakfast: Green Bean Almondine
- Lunch: Caribbean Chicken Stew
- Dinner: Chicken Stuffed Bell Peppers

Day 3:
- Breakfast: Roasted Turnips with Parsley
- Lunch: Lentil and Spinach Soup
- Dinner: Chicken Fajitas

Day 4:
- Breakfast: Stir-fried Bok Choy
- Lunch: Split Pea Soup
- Dinner: Lemon and Thyme Turkey Cutlets

Day 5:
- Breakfast: Vegetarian Chili
- Lunch: White Bean and Kale Soup
- Dinner: Pan-Seared Tuna Steaks

Day 6:
- Breakfast: Asparagus Lemon Pasta
- Lunch: Italian Sausage and Potato Soup
- Dinner: Broiled Snapper with Tomato Relish

Day 7:
- Breakfast: Cabbage Slaw with Honey Lime Dressing
- Lunch: Barley and Mushroom Soup
- Dinner: Cajun Catfish with Sweet Potato Mash

Week 6
Day 1:
- Breakfast: Sautéed Swiss Chard with Pine Nuts
- Lunch: Turkey and Sweet Potato Hash
- Dinner: Mediterranean Baked Sardines

Day 2:
- Breakfast: Asparagus Lemon Pasta
- Lunch: Chicken Tortilla Soup
- Dinner: Scallops with Pea Puree

Day 3:
- Breakfast: Vegetarian Chili
- Lunch: White Bean and Kale Soup
- Dinner: Broiled Snapper with Tomato Relish

Day 4:
- Breakfast: Cabbage Slaw with Honey Lime Dressing
- Lunch: Barley and Mushroom Soup
- Dinner: Cajun Catfish with Sweet Potato Mash

Day 5:
- Breakfast: Spaghetti Squash Primavera
- Lunch: Sweet Potato and Red Lentil Soup
- Dinner: Herb-Crusted Sole

Day 6:
- Breakfast: Roasted Radishes with Rosemary
- Lunch: Caribbean Chicken Stew
- Dinner: Chicken and Spinach Curry

Day 7:
- Breakfast: Eggplant Caponata
- Lunch: Lentil and Spinach Soup
- Dinner: Chicken and Vegetable Kebabs

Week 7
Day 1:
- Breakfast: Roasted Brussels Sprouts with Garlic
- Lunch: Italian Sausage and Potato Soup
- Dinner: Pan-Seared Tuna Steaks

Day 2:
- Breakfast: Green Bean Almondine
- Lunch: Caribbean Chicken Stew
- Dinner: Chicken Stuffed Bell Peppers

Day 3:
- Breakfast: Roasted Turnips with Parsley
- Lunch: Lentil and Spinach Soup
- Dinner: Chicken Fajitas

Day 4:
- Breakfast: Stir-fried Bok Choy
- Lunch: Split Pea Soup
- Dinner: Lemon and Thyme Turkey Cutlets

Day 5:
- Breakfast: Vegetarian Chili
- Lunch: White Bean and Kale Soup
- Dinner: Pan-Seared Tuna Steaks

Day 6:
- Breakfast: Asparagus Lemon Pasta
- Lunch: Italian Sausage and Potato Soup
- Dinner: Broiled Snapper with Tomato Relish

Day 7:
- Breakfast: Cabbage Slaw with Honey Lime Dressing
- Lunch: Barley and Mushroom Soup
- Dinner: Cajun Catfish with Sweet Potato Mash

Week 8

Day 1:
- Breakfast: Spaghetti Squash Primavera
- Lunch: Sweet Potato and Red Lentil Soup
- Dinner: Herb-Crusted Sole

Day 2:
- Breakfast: Roasted Radishes with Rosemary
- Lunch: Caribbean Chicken Stew
- Dinner: Chicken and Spinach Curry

Day 3:
- Breakfast: Eggplant Caponata
- Lunch: Lentil and Spinach Soup
- Dinner: Chicken and Vegetable Kebabs

Day 4:
- Breakfast: Grilled Eggplant with Tomato and Basil
- Lunch: Chicken Tortilla Soup
- Dinner: Turkey Meatballs in Marinara Sauce

Day 5:
- Breakfast: Green Bean Almondine
- Lunch: Spicy Black Bean Soup
- Dinner: Chicken Fajitas

Day 6:
- Breakfast: Cabbage Slaw with Honey Lime Dressing
- Lunch: Italian Sausage and Potato Soup
- Dinner: Lemon Butter Haddock

Day 7:
- Breakfast: Spaghetti Squash Primavera
- Lunch: White Bean and Kale Soup
- Dinner: Broiled Snapper with Tomato Relish

Week 9

Day 1:
- Breakfast: Roasted Turnips with Parsley
- Lunch: Sweet Potato and Red Lentil Soup
- Dinner: Scallops with Pea Puree

Day 2:
- Breakfast: Stir-fried Bok Choy
- Lunch: Barley and Mushroom Soup
- Dinner: Cajun Catfish with Sweet Potato Mash

Day 3:
- Breakfast: Vegetarian Chili
- Lunch: Caribbean Chicken Stew
- Dinner: Pan-Seared Tuna Steaks

Day 4:
- Breakfast: Cabbage Slaw with Honey Lime Dressing
- Lunch: Italian Sausage and Potato Soup
- Dinner: Broiled Snapper with Tomato Relish

Day 5:
- Breakfast: Green Bean Almondine
- Lunch: White Bean and Kale Soup
- Dinner: Lemon Butter Haddock

Day 6:
- Breakfast: Eggplant Caponata
- Lunch: Lentil and Spinach Soup
- Dinner: Chicken and Vegetable Kebabs

Day 7:
- Breakfast: Grilled Eggplant with Tomato and Basil
- Lunch: Chicken Tortilla Soup
- Dinner: Turkey Meatballs in Marinara Sauce

Week 10

Day 1:
- Breakfast: Spaghetti Squash Primavera
- Lunch: Sweet Potato and Red Lentil Soup
- Dinner: Herb-Crusted Sole

Day 2:
- Breakfast: Roasted Radishes with Rosemary
- Lunch: Caribbean Chicken Stew
- Dinner: Chicken and Spinach Curry

Day 3:
- Breakfast: Eggplant Caponata
- Lunch: Lentil and Spinach Soup
- Dinner: Chicken and Vegetable Kebabs

Day 4:
- Breakfast: Green Bean Almondine
- Lunch: Barley and Mushroom Soup
- Dinner: Cajun Catfish with Sweet Potato Mash

Day 5:
- Breakfast: Vegetarian Chili
- Lunch: White Bean and Kale Soup
- Dinner: Lemon Butter Haddock

Day 6:
- Breakfast: Cabbage Slaw with Honey Lime Dressing
- Lunch: Italian Sausage and Potato Soup
- Dinner: Broiled Snapper with Tomato Relish

Day 7:
- Breakfast: Grilled Eggplant with Tomato and Basil
- Lunch: Chicken Tortilla Soup
- Dinner: Turkey Meatballs in Marinara Sauce

Weekly Meal planner + Journal

	BREAKFAST	LUNCH	DINNER	SNACKS
MON				
TUE				
WED				
THU				
FRI				
SAT				
SUN				

Why are you interested in starting the LIPEDEMA diet? Reflect on your motivations and goals for adopting this diet.

....

....

....

....

....

....

....

Weekly Meal planner + Journal

	BREAKFAST	LUNCH	DINNER	SNACKS
MON				
TUE				
WED				
THU				
FRI				
SAT				
SUN				

What symptoms of LIPEDEMA are you currently experiencing? List your symptoms and how they affect your daily life.

....
....
....
....
....
....
....

Weekly Meal planner + Journal

	BREAKFAST	LUNCH	DINNER	SNACKS
MON				
TUE				
WED				
THU				
FRI				
SAT				
SUN				

How do you feel about making dietary changes to manage your LIPEDEMA? Consider your emotions and readiness for this lifestyle change.

....

....

....

....

....

....

....

Weekly Meal planner + Journal

	BREAKFAST	LUNCH	DINNER	SNACKS
MON				
TUE				
WED				
THU				
FRI				
SAT				
SUN				

What challenges do you anticipate when starting the LIPEDEMA diet? Think about potential obstacles and how you might overcome them.

....
....
....
....
....
....
....

Weekly Meal planner + Journal

	BREAKFAST	LUNCH	DINNER	SNACKS
MON				
TUE				
WED				
THU				
FRI				
SAT				
SUN				

What strategies can you use to stay hydrated throughout the day? Develop a plan to ensure you drink enough water and fluids.

....

....

....

....

....

....

....

Weekly Meal planner + Journal

	BREAKFAST	LUNCH	DINNER	SNACKS
MON				
TUE				
WED				
THU				
FRI				
SAT				
SUN				

How will you ensure you avoid foods that exacerbate LIPEDEMA symptoms? Identify foods to avoid and create a plan to eliminate them from your diet.

....

....

....

....

....

....

....

Weekly Meal planner + Journal

	BREAKFAST	LUNCH	DINNER	SNACKS
MON				
TUE				
WED				
THU				
FRI				
SAT				
SUN				

What support systems do you have in place to help you with this dietary change? List friends, family, or healthcare professionals who can support you.

....
....
....
....
....
....
....

Weekly Meal planner + Journal

	BREAKFAST	LUNCH	DINNER	SNACKS
MON				
TUE				
WED				
THU				
FRI				
SAT				
SUN				

What are your short-term and long-term goals for managing LIPEDEMA through diet? Set achievable goals and milestones for your dietary journey.

....

....

....

....

....

....

....

Weekly Meal planner + Journal

	BREAKFAST	LUNCH	DINNER	SNACKS
MON				
TUE				
WED				
THU				
FRI				
SAT				
SUN				

How will you handle social situations or dining out while following the LIPEDEMA diet? Plan strategies for sticking to your diet in social settings.

....

....

....

....

....

....

....

Weekly Meal planner + Journal

	BREAKFAST	LUNCH	DINNER	SNACKS
MON				
TUE				
WED				
THU				
FRI				
SAT				
SUN				

What questions or concerns do you have about starting the LIPEDEMA diet? List any uncertainties and plan to discuss them with your healthcare provider.

....

....

....

....

....

....

....

Scan the QR code below to get a surprise bonus

www.ingramcontent.com/pod-product-compliance
Lightning Source LLC
Chambersburg PA
CBHW082234220526
45479CB00005B/1233